"De Loof skillfully guides the reader through conversations with Slootmaeckers and Migerode that offer a unique and helpful perspective on partner violence that is a great asset for all types of couples struggling with escalating conflict that ends in violence. While intended as a self-help book, it is also a terrific resource for therapists. By presenting love and violence as two sides of the same coin, they counter the taboo of speaking about situational partner violence and the shame of continuing to love someone who deeply hurts them physically and emotionally. They shift common, scrutinizing questions of, 'What is wrong with you? with me? with us?' to the nonjudgmental question of, 'What is happening between us?'

They openly acknowledge the influence of Johnson's attachment-oriented emotionally focused therapy (EFT) model, as they reframe the stigma-laden language of *perpetrator, victim, power-seeking and anger issues* to the attachment-oriented view of *aggression as contact-seeking or distance-seeking behaviors* stuck in repeating cycles of pain and powerlessness. Providing language to talk safely about partner violence, they describe vividly and compassionately how a loving connection can turn into cycles of pain.

The book paves a path of safety to talk openly about partner violence for those experiencing it first hand while isolating in a pressure cooker of shame and fear. While consistently finding the goodness in partners whose behavior has gotten out of control, and highlighting couples' desire to stop the violence, Jef and Lieven provide an indispensable guidebook for partners willing to take responsibility to stop violent escalations. This is a vital resource to help partners to experience violence as a wake-up call to *work together* toward change to achieve the interpersonal safety, security, and connection they desire."

Lorrie Brubacher, M.Ed., LMFT, author of *Stepping into Emotionally Focused Therapy: Key Ingredients of Change*, 2nd ed., (Routledge, 2025), Adjunct, UNC Greensboro, NC, EFT Trainer http://www.dkceft.dk/

"This book is a must read for anyone interested in better understanding the emotional and relational undercurrent that can lead to escalating arguments and violence in relationships, the aftermath that follows, and the path home, from disconnection to connection. With the wisdom gleaned from their shared table, their therapy spaces, and beyond, Jef and Lieven offer readers a close up look at a topic that is often hidden. Woven throughout this book are excerpts of their dialogue, stories of people grappling with the scars of violence in relationships, and, most importantly, answers to the key questions that offer compassion, care, and clarity. Whether you are a therapist, a client, or someone searching for the answers to your own proclivity to react rather than reach during times of interpersonal threat, perceived danger, or loss, this beautifully written and accessible book will most certainly prove a trustworthy companion and guide out of helplessness and defeat into hope and resilience. Most certainly, if you or someone you know is caught in the throes of disconnection and fighting for connection, this book will provide a much-needed perspective. Highly recommended!"

Dr. T. Leanne Campbell, Registered Psychologist and ICEEFT Executive Board Member

"*How can two people love each other deeply and still hurt each other so profoundly?* This question sits at the center of this book, which offers a thoughtful and compassionate way of understanding partner violence without reducing it to blame or pathology. Rather than asking what is 'wrong' with one partner or the other, the authors keep the focus where it belongs: on what happens between two people in an intimate relationship when fear, longing, and loss of connection collide.

One of the book's great strengths is how clearly it situates partner violence within the context of attachment and escalation. Many couples describe the painful realization that they have 'crossed a line' they never wanted to cross. The authors treat this moment not as proof that love is absent, but as a signal that something essential has broken down in the relationship's ability to regulate intense emotion. Violence, in this framing, is not separate from love; it often emerges from its rupture.

The distinction between *hot* and *cold* partner violence is especially useful. Cold violence, one-sided and instrumental, is what most people imagine when they hear the term, but it is relatively rare. Far more common is hot violence, which unfolds in relationships marked by emotional closeness, mutual vulnerability, and unresolved attachment pain. Naming this difference allows for greater clarity, responsibility, and more accurate clinical understanding.

The authors' use of the 'Finally!' moment, the sense of arrival and belonging that accompanies falling in love, beautifully captures why conflict can hurt so much. Love answers deep questions: *Am I good enough? Are you there for me? Do I belong?* When those questions are threatened, the pain can feel overwhelming. Partners respond by moving toward each other or pulling away and this familiar dance can escalate until words are no longer enough. The book helps readers see how quickly attachment fear can take over and how easily it can tip into destructive behavior.

The authors are also honest about why it is so hard to talk about partner violence. People are told to speak up, yet also hear that violence is dangerous, forbidden, and shameful. Many couples become stuck between fear of consequences, fear of escalation, and fear of how they will be judged. Shame plays a central role here, shaping responses such as withdrawal, attack, self-blame, or avoidance. At the same time, the book captures the relief that can come when vulnerable feelings are finally spoken and met with presence rather than rejection.

The impact on children is addressed with care and realism. Asking whether conflict is harming one's children is framed as a sign of concern, not failure. While parents cannot undo what has already happened, they can acknowledge it, talk about it, and reassure their children that safety and repair matter. This simple but powerful shift can ease fear and interrupt the repetition of painful patterns across generations.

Importantly, the book challenges the belief that once violence appears, it inevitably worsens. Research and clinical experience suggest otherwise. Many couples do stop the violence, especially when they learn to recognize escalation earlier and take responsibility together for changing how they fight. The authors make clear that lasting change does not happen when one is alone, but it happens in a relationship.

This is not a book of quick solutions. It is a grounded, humane guide for couples and clinicians willing to face painful dynamics with honesty, care, and hope. I highly recommend it to anyone committed to helping relationships move toward greater safety, responsibility, and connection."

Jette Sinkjær Simon, Clinical Psychologist, Specialist in Psychotherapy and Supervision, Director of the Danish Center for Emotionally Focused Therapy

Fighting for Connection

Fighting for Connection offers a fresh, nuanced perspective on conflict and partner violence, blending emotional, relational, and scientific insights through the lens of Emotionally Focused Therapy (EFT). This book speaks to couples experiencing escalating conflict, as well as to professionals supporting them. It moves beyond traditional narratives of power or victimhood to explore the emotional and relational dynamics that underlie violent interactions.

Structured as a conversation between two experts in EFT and domestic violence, the authors answer the questions couples often ask themselves when caught in cycles of escalation. Readers are guided through the complexities of love, conflict, and emotional pain, engaging with the material in an accessible, empathetic style. This book combines clear explanations with research-based insights, while ensuring the language resonates with lived experiences.

With its original dual audience approach, it speaks directly to couples living through high-conflict situations and simultaneously equips therapists, counselors, and social workers with practical frameworks and strategies rooted in EFT. It reframes partner violence as a relational problem, providing pathways toward healing without oversimplifying the challenges involved. Through real-world examples, therapy principles, and actionable guidance, this book empowers readers to restore safety, connection, and empathy in relationships.

Jef Slootmaeckers, LMFT, is the director of EFT-Belgium and a certified EFT therapist, supervisor, and trainer. He specializes in working with intimate partner violence, trauma, shame, and aggression. Jef delivers EFT and violence trainings internationally.

Lieven Migerode, C.Psych., MFT, is the founder of EFT-Belgium and a certified EFT therapist, supervisor, and trainer emeritus. With 40 years of couples therapy experience, he co-teaches EFT and violence with Jef Slootmaeckers and has published several books and articles on love and partner violence.

Linne De Loof is a clinical psychologist, contextual systemic therapist, and EFT therapist and supervisor. She works with individuals, families, and especially couples, helping them in their quest for a safe connection. Her interest in human dynamics and passion for language is reflected in several publications and books.

Fighting for Connection

Perspectives on Conflict and Intimate Partner Violence

JEF SLOOTMAECKERS, LIEVEN MIGERODE, AND LINNE DE LOOF

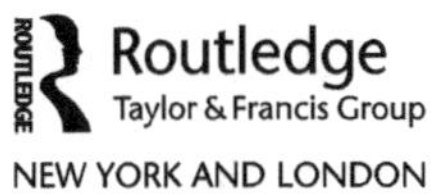

NEW YORK AND LONDON

Designed cover image: Getty Images

First published in English 2027
by Routledge
605 Third Avenue, New York, NY 10158

and by Routledge
4 Park Square, Milton Park, Abingdon, Oxon, OX14 4RN

Routledge is an imprint of the Taylor & Francis Group, an informa business

Published in Dutch by Pelckmans 2024

Translated by DeepL and edited by Jef Slootmaeckers, Lieven Migerode and Linne De Loof

Library of Congress Cataloging-in-Publication Data
A catalog record for this title has been requested

ISBN: 978-1-041-16255-1 (hbk)
ISBN: 978-1-041-16173-8 (pbk)
ISBN: 978-1-003-68358-2 (ebk)

DOI: 10.4324/9781003683582

Typeset in Dante MT Std
by codeMantra

Contents

Acknowledgments

A heartfelt thank you to all the couples who entrusted us with their stories.

It is an honor to serve as the megaphone for your wisdom in this book.

INTRODUCTION

The birth of a story about partner violence

Welcome to *Fighting for Love.*

This book is authored by Jef Slootmaeckers and Lieven Migerode, both experts in the complex intersection of love and violence. Before we explore their insights, we would like to introduce these two professionals, explain for whom this book was written, describe how it came to be, and outline the context that informs it. Jef and Lieven are both couples therapists who have been working together on the topic of partner violence for nearly a decade. Yet even before they met, this issue had already connected their professional paths.

From meeting to collaboration

Jef has long been fascinated by intimate relationships and the phenomenon of partner violence. His professional involvement began almost 20 years ago. After several years of working with people experiencing homelessness, he transitioned to a shelter—a facility for women and children fleeing partner violence. He later joined the first team in Flanders offering relationship therapy to couples affected by the very same violence he had encountered in the shelter setting.

DOI: 10.4324/9781003683582-1

Lieven: "Jef was never just doing his job as a social worker. From the start, he was thinking deeply about the problem. He noticed that 70% of the women who came to the shelter eventually returned to their partners, despite the prevailing approach being focused on breaking off the relationship and encouraging the women to move on independently. That made him wonder: How can we understand this phenomenon? And what does it mean for the support we offer these women, their partners, and their children? He wasn't just thinking—he started writing about it. At one point, he sent his writing to me. In it, I found true insight into how we might understand something as complex as partner violence. His perspective was far more nuanced and open than the usual judgmental narrative. That was the beginning of an intense collaboration that eventually led to the book you now hold."

Jef: "Yes, I sort of stumbled into this field, but it grabbed me right away, and I couldn't let it go. The dominant discourse around partner violence focused heavily on power and control, but I found that framework lacking in my day-to-day work at the shelter. In many cases, it simply didn't align with what I was witnessing. As I searched for new ways to understand partner violence, I came across Lieven's work. At our first meeting, I thought, *'Goddamn, asshole!'* Let me explain—he's a kind man! I had read a chapter on partner violence he had co-authored with Geertje Walraevens (Migerode & Walravens, 2011) and it included this sentence: *'Could it not be that love and violence are two sides of the same coin?'* I was both startled and frustrated. I had written that exact sentence in my own notes just weeks earlier, but Lieven had published it, and I hadn't. After a few weeks of grumbling, I realized this shouldn't be an ending but a beginning. I needed to talk to this man who seemed to think about partner violence the same way I did."

At the time, Lieven had over 30 years of experience working with couples at the University Psychiatric Center KU Leuven and in private practice and had been focused on partner violence since 1998. Many couples affected by violence approached a therapist, only to be turned away with the message: "Come back when there's no more violence." Lieven fought to create space within the therapeutic landscape for these couples, with all their struggles and suffering. That shared struggle brought Jef and Lieven together. They began collaborating—debating, analyzing, writing, and sharing experiences—and they haven't stopped since.

For a long time, Lieven had sensed that love was missing from the discourse in couples therapy. It may sound strange, but until recently, love had been an underexplored theme in the field. Inspired by the work of Sue Johnson, who reframed love as attachment within the framework of Emotionally Focused Therapy (EFT), Lieven began to write about it and eventually brought EFT to

Belgium. In 2014, he led the country's first major EFT training. Jef was one of the participants. From that moment, they shared a common language for talking about relationships. Over time, they deepened their understanding of EFT's core concepts—love, attachment, emotion, and interaction—and began applying them to another underrepresented theme in couples therapy: partner violence.

Lieven: "At that point, I had all but given up on trying to introduce an approach to partner violence grounded in love. Years earlier, I had traveled to Slovenia to attend workshops by Sandra Stith, a leading expert in the field. We shared a common vision, but it never took root in Belgium. Meeting Jef changed that. He brought firsthand experience with violent couples, and I brought insights from love-centered couples therapy. EFT became the bridge connecting our perspectives. From then on, we spent years in dialogue: reviewing each other's work, co-authoring articles, and giving trainings together."

EFT as a backdrop

As you'll notice throughout this introduction, and increasingly throughout the book, Jef and Lieven frequently reference EFT. While not the central focus of the book, it forms the conceptual foundation for their approach. So, a brief explanation is in order. EFT, developed by Sue Johnson, is a relatively recent therapy model that has become one of the most thoroughly researched in the field, particularly in couples therapy. It is also applied to individuals and families. EFT views relational tensions as cycles of interaction—something we will explore in detail later in the book—rooted in the need for secure emotional attachment. This model places love at the forefront, positing that our protective responses to emotional insecurity often entrench us in recurring patterns of behavior. EFT follows a clear sequence: first, we must understand what is happening between partners before we can address it. The goal is to foster a relationship environment in which both partners can share their inner emotional world and be received with empathy, creating greater emotional safety.

Jef: "EFT is a model in which Lieven and I immediately recognized essential truths, not only for ourselves and those close to us but also for the people we work with. From our very first exposure, we were captivated. No other therapeutic approach had ever so accurately reflected what we were seeing in practice. We immersed ourselves in the model: we became certified EFT therapists, then supervisors, and eventually trainers. And even now, it continues to fascinate us. EFT isn't a model where you have to memorize abstract concepts or imagine how they apply: it aligns directly with real-life experiences. For us as therapists, it offers a coherent and logical framework to follow. At the same time, it requires experience and, most importantly, attunement to adapt the model to the specific couple sitting in front of you. In that sense, EFT is our map, but it's the couples who show us the landscape. And that landscape looks different every time."

A quirky take on partner violence

In developing their approach to partner violence and couple therapy, Lieven and Jef combined two guiding principles: bottom-up and top-down thinking. On the one hand, they spent considerable time discussing and reflecting on each other's clinical work with couples experiencing violence. Most importantly, they listened deeply to what these couples were telling them. "What wisdom do these people hold, and how can we respond appropriately through counseling and therapy?" they asked. At the same time, they immersed themselves in international research on partner violence and escalating conflict. These two perspectives—practice and theory—converged to produce a unique and innovative way of working with partner violence.

They found significant inspiration in EFT. However, they applied this model to a population historically excluded from EFT practices and, more broadly, from most forms of couples therapy. Until recently, partner violence was widely considered a contraindication for couples therapy. Lieven and Jef, however, shared the conviction that this did not need to be the case. Their thesis is bold: not only is couples therapy possible in cases of partner violence, but it may, in fact, be the most appropriate therapeutic response for couples caught in cycles of escalating conflict.

Their novel approach attracted attention, and they were soon invited to present and teach it around the world. Again and again, they encountered therapists and social workers who, after attending their training, expressed a sense of relief: they finally had language for something they had long intuited—that partner violence and escalation are, in many cases, desperate expressions of a fight for love. That core insight is the heart of this book.

Jef: "In 2018, we were sitting at a sidewalk café near the station square in Leuven when I said to Lieven, 'We have to write a book. We need to articulate our perspective on partner violence—not for therapists, but for people who experience it firsthand, people who are struggling.' Lieven replied, 'Well, I'd like to write about that.' So, we began. But once we started writing, we realized we first needed to describe the therapeutic process to explain what we were doing. Before we knew it, we had written a book for therapists (Slootmaeckers & Migerode, 2026). We thought, 'Now we'll never write again,' since we're both dyslexic, and writing a book is something of a torture for us. But the idea wouldn't let go."

The people Lieven and Jef work for are those who suffer through relationship escalations and seek help. Research shows that individuals dealing with partner violence often first turn to written resources in their search for understanding. Yet, very few of these sources convey the presence of love within the conflict. That absence continued to trouble them. Eventually, they reached out for help—help with writing.

Jef: "It so happens that my partner is not only a wonderful wife and mother but also a skilled couples therapist and an excellent writer. Linne De Loof is deeply familiar with working with violent couples and with our vision. She had already written several pieces that Lieven and I admired. She felt a strong resonance with these ideas and wanted to help put them into words. Thanks to her, the original concept of the book has finally taken shape."

Writing by, for, and about couples in conflict

This book is written, first and foremost, for people who are themselves suffering from partner violence. It is intended for all couples who are grappling with conflicts, whether mild or extreme, who want to understand what is happening, and who yearn to approach it differently. Second, the book addresses those close to such couples—family, friends, or professionals—who are also affected by the tensions and want to better comprehend this complex phenomenon. Finally, therapists and counselors may find valuable insights here into the inner world of couples locked in conflict but still striving for love.

Lieven: "This book is not just for those who are painfully and confusingly caught in the cycle of loving each other and yet physically hurting one another. It's also for those who want to understand how relationships work—how recurring conflict patterns function—and who want to learn more about love through its struggles. We want to offer hope to anyone searching for it in their relationships. While the book does explore extreme moments when things go badly wrong, those moments are often preceded by the small, everyday frustrations and interactions. So, it's also a book for people who repeatedly run into the same issues in their relationships. In short, this book is for couples dealing with both the small and the large conflicts."

This book is meant to complement the many excellent works that already exist on partner violence. Most current writing, however, focuses on one specific form: intimate terrorism—also known as coercive controlling violence—a term widely used in the literature. Intimate terrorism involves instrumental, controlling violence in which there is a clear perpetrator and a clear victim. We explain this further in the book. In short, this form of aggression is rooted in power and domination, with little or no presence of love. Understandably, this form of violence has received much attention. Yet, there are two recognized forms of partner violence: intimate terrorism and situational couple violence. The latter arises from escalating conflict between partners who genuinely care about each other. Situational couple violence is, by far, the more common type. This is well documented across a broad base of international research. And yet, very little has been written about it, especially in ways that are accessible to the general public.

Jef: "With this book, we want to extend a warm welcome to all people who live with partner violence but do not recognize themselves in the often-horrific image associated with intimate terrorism. The group we are addressing is far larger than society tends to acknowledge. These are not perpetrators and victims in the traditional sense, but people who are trying to build a safe home together and find themselves stuck. Explaining exactly how that happens—that's what this book is for. So, the book is intended for couples who are experiencing partner violence, who still love one another, and who are looking for more compassionate, constructive ways to handle the tensions they face."

The questions from him/her/them/...

Over the past several years, Lieven and Jef have encountered a series of recurring questions in their work with couples suffering from violence in their relationships: *How is it possible that we love each other so much and still hurt each other this deeply? Is what happens between us considered partner violence? What exactly is going on between us that things can spiral so far out of control? If it gets this bad, does that mean something is wrong with me? With my partner? With us as a couple? Why is it still so hard to talk about this, especially with each other but also with those around us? Are these escalating conflicts harming our children? Will this destructive cycle ever come to an end?*

These are the kinds of questions that emerge in nearly every relationship where things have gotten out of hand. And it is precisely these questions that this book seeks to explore and clarify. Lieven and Jef have had—and continue to have—the privilege of speaking and working with hundreds of couples who know partner violence from the inside out. These couples have taught them what is at stake and how to better understand what unfolds in such relationships. Through these encounters, the two therapists have been able to take steps toward finding answers. This book is, in that sense, a preliminary reflection of what Jef and Lieven have learned from couples about these urgent and deeply human questions.

It was with these seven questions in mind that Linne approached Lieven and Jef. They sat down together at a table, and Linne posed each question one by one, inviting open conversation, just as they would when co-developing a concept or leading a training session. Each chapter of this book is a representation of one of those conversations. At times, the dialogue focused on conceptualizing partner violence; at other moments, it explored their therapeutic practice. Sometimes the emphasis was on what they "know"; at other times, the uncertainty and searching were more palpable. At times the therapists spoke; at other times, they gave the floor to the voices of the couples themselves.

Lieven: "When we refer to 'couples' in this book, we mean all forms of intimate partnerships where two people love each other—woman–woman, man–woman, man–man; cisgender, transgender, or non-binary; individuals questioning their sexual orientation or gender identity who are nonetheless in a relationship. Any 'she' you read could just as easily be a 'he' or 'they,' and vice versa. Our goal is to welcome everyone and every form of relationship. In writing this book, we have strived to honor this diversity, but we are aware that we have inevitably fallen short. The same applies to other forms of diversity. Although we are Flemish authors, this book extends its welcome to couples worldwide—multicultural couples, couples from immigrant backgrounds, and more. This theme—relationship violence—is profoundly universal. It cuts across all walks of life, all (sub)cultures, and all kinds of relational forms. No matter how inclusively we aim to write, we will miss people, overlook nuances, and bypass specific forms of injustice or exclusion. We acknowledge this. What we can do is share that our intention, always, is to welcome everyone."

With this extended welcome, we have laid the groundwork for the framework surrounding this book. Now it's time to enter the heart of the matter: the questions that arise when conflict begins to take the wheel in your relationship. And so we begin with the first and foundational question: 'Is this partner violence?'

We wish you a meaningful and courageous reading experience—and above all, strength and confidence in your journey toward fighting more lovingly.

References

Migerode, L., & Walravens, G. (2011). Een visie op liefde en geweld bij koppels. In A. Groenen, E. Jaspaert, & G. Vervaeke (Eds.), *Partnergeweld - Als liefde een gevecht wordt.* (pp. 115–127). Acco.

Slootmaeckers, J., & Migerode, M. (2026). *Partner violence and emotionally focused therapy: Fighting for love.* RJPi.

1
IS THIS PARTNER VIOLENCE?

To talk about relationships is also to talk about quarrels. People in relationships share joy, find support and peace with one another, and enjoy their time together. At the same time, these same people clash, tensions build, differences cause distance, and arguments arise. Sometimes these quarrels escalate—more intensely in some couples than in others. Occasionally, the conflict really spirals out of control. This can range from persistent, hurtful criticism and intense outbursts of swearing or humiliating remarks, to silent treatment lasting days, to sexual boundary violations or physical outbursts involving broken objects, pushing, pulling, or even severe blows that leave partners injured. People caught in such escalating tensions often ask themselves: "Is this partner violence? What exactly is partner violence? At what point do we say it's partner violence? Does it have to involve physical acts, or does it also include blaming and hurtful words?" These are important questions, revealing how deeply people suffer in such situations. These questions arise not only among couples themselves but also among social workers and others in their environment.

DOI: 10.4324/9781003683582-2

The risk of a definition

When we answer the question, "Is this partner violence?" we deliberately avoid starting with a strict definition. Instead, we begin with the stories of people we meet in therapy and gradually develop a description of the complex reality of partner violence. We outline what we understand from the experiences of couples caught in this dynamic. We do not provide a simple "yes" or "no" answer. Above all, we want to offer a welcoming space to all who struggle with escalating conflicts. As you read on, we invite you into this book and into your own search to understand what happens in and between partners in conflict.

Jef: "I remember a phone call I received recently. A man called me, speaking very hesitantly—and soon I understood why. He told me that he cared deeply for his partner, but that they argued a lot—sometimes fiercely. So fiercely, in fact, that just last week, his partner ended up in the hospital. He had pushed her, and she fell, hitting her head on the edge of a glass coffee table, leaving a deep wound. Very quietly, he said, 'I just don't understand how that could happen, because we really love each other. It all happened so fast… I don't want this to ever happen again, so that's why I'd like to make an appointment with you. I read online that you had written about partner violence, and I think that's what's going on with us. Can we meet? Or is what happened at our place too serious?' The tension was palpable in his voice.

Partner violence is very common, yet rarely spoken about. As a result, people often don't know exactly what it is or how to understand it. With this book, we want to create space for those questions. And so we start at the beginning: what is partner violence? We choose to keep the question, 'Is this partner violence?' intentionally broad. There are many definitions of partner violence. Type it into Google, and you'll find a long list, some more nuanced than others. But I hesitate to start there… *Definitions often overlook nuances and tend to invite judgment*: What is acceptable? What is not? And judgment is precisely what conflict dynamics feed on. We want to avoid stepping into those dynamics here.

Couples often explain this better than I can. Yesterday, a couple sat with me. The wife described how they had gotten caught up in another conflict last weekend. She said, 'This time was really bad. He crossed a line. It started as usual: I was managing everything—the kids, the hobbies, the dog, errands... carrying the entire household on my shoulders, cleaning up messes and problems... and he didn't even notice. No, he was reading his newspaper. When I saw him step over the neatly folded laundry on the stairs for the third time that day, something snapped. I was so disappointed, exhausted, and furious. I told him how I felt. Do you know what he did next? He slapped me in the face. Like I was a child. Can you imagine that, Jef? I'm struggling like that, I open my soul, and then he just attacks me.' She turned her head to the side and pointed to a blue mark near her ear. 'That's pure aggression, isn't it? That's violence, isn't it, Jef? You really can't do that anymore!' Her desperation was clear.

Before I could respond, her husband interrupted bitterly, 'That's what you call violence?!' He laughed harshly. 'Then what did you do? You started screaming and shouting that I'm worthless, a zero, that no woman in the world deserves me... in front of our daughter. Who's being aggressive here? Do you know what that does to me? You took the laundry down the stairs and threw it around, tore my shirt in two right before my eyes—you don't tell Jef about that. So, who is violent? I agree I shouldn't have hit you. But when all I hear is how worthless I am, that nothing I do matters to you... there's nothing left of me. All I wanted was for you to stop with those humiliating insults.'

Do you feel how difficult it is in this situation to say what counts as partner violence? We want to take the time to answer this question with nuance."

Lieven: "Indeed, partner violence cannot be easily defined. I imagine readers may wonder, 'What is happening with us? What can we call it?' There are many possible answers. Jef's first response is a caution: 'Be careful with that question because it can become just another way of fighting.' Words can be used to hurt, just like blows. That would undermine the purpose of this book—to help you handle tension and conflict more constructively.

What we want to focus on here is this: Sometimes painful situations in relationships lead, whether together or separately, to physical or excessively violent verbal arguments. An experience where you feel, '*This crosses a line*. This is not what we want.' We assume that those people say, 'Darn, it's bad for us that we end up here.' That is what this book addresses. That is how we understand partner violence."

Jef: "Our hesitation to respond directly to the question, 'Is this partner violence?' comes from the fact that such an answer can provoke further conflict. Let me illustrate. When I worked at the Social Services Centre I worked one day a week at reception. People came in voluntarily, with all kinds of questions. For example, one day, a woman came to me and said, 'I had an argument with my partner yesterday and it got out of hand. I saw a TV report on partner violence, and I recognize that in us.' At that moment, you have two options. You can ask her, 'What exactly happened? How did it happen? What did your partner do? What did you do?' Then you could apply a definition and decide, 'Yes, this qualifies as partner violence.' Later, that woman might go home, sit at the kitchen table, and say to her partner, 'What you did yesterday—that's violence. The man at the CAW said so.' I don't think the conversation at the kitchen table will be calm. It's interesting to consider what effect this has. I worry it will escalate the conflict because the situation is being defined one-sidedly. The partner might feel the need to defend themselves, which will increase tension and relational conflict. I don't know if the woman would actually feel helped by that.

What we can do instead is say, 'Welcome. It seems like your relationship—and what's happening in it—is really important to you. So important that you came here to talk to me, a complete stranger. It seems like you want to understand what's going on between you. Let's look together at what's happening between you in those moments, shall we?' Then we shift from 'What is it?' to 'What is happening between you?' and 'What exactly brings you here?' I assume that beneath it lies an experience of lost love. This hurts deeply and at the same time creates a longing. That longing is a crucial motivation to face these issues. I think this is true for the readers of this book as well. So, welcome to the longing for love that brings you here."

Answering a complex issue like partner violence with a simple answer risks losing nuance and introducing judgment. Judgment often fuels new conflict. Therefore, we choose to start from the whole experience of people caught up in it. This leads us to an important description couples give: they have "crossed the line." They feel they have crossed a boundary they did not want to cross. This appears to be a key element in understanding partner violence.

"We don't want this!"

The term *partner violence* often carries a heavy connotation of judgment, something definitive. In public discourse, partner violence is frequently linked with condemnation. The topic is highly polarized. Words like *perpetrator* and *victim* immediately arise. These words are not used in this book. Yet, we do not want to ignore the pain, damage, or violence involved. Searching for a balanced answer to the initial question reveals how difficult it is to discuss this topic without falling into extremes or opposites.

Lieven: "Although we don't start with a strict definition, we do move toward some kind of description. After all, it is helpful to say, 'This is violence.' Take the example of the woman at the reception you mentioned. She recognizes, 'This is partner violence.' She is aware of the social meanings attached to the term and wonders, 'Should I look at myself and my relationship differently? I'm asking for help.' The danger in stating categorically, 'This is partner violence' or 'This is not,' is that one partner may feel unseen, which can increase conflict or even violence. So this is a caution for counselors—and readers alike: don't use the definition of violence to 'hit' your partner over the head. I understand that completely.

At the same time, something happens during escalation that has distinct characteristics. People themselves say, 'We don't want this. It's a way of relating to each other that we reject—and we might call that violence.' People experiencing this often—obviously influenced by societal views—arrive at some form of definition on their own. To that, I also say, 'Welcome.'

Something emerges in relationships that people do not want: something they say, do, or call out. To quote Jef, 'Very few people wake up thinking, "I'm going to hit my partner hard today."' That is truly rare, and we will discuss it later. Yet, when two people are calm and connected, you see very little yelling, pulling, hitting, biting, spitting, or cursing. That tells you something about what partner violence really is.

It arises between people who live together and share a relationship. *Tension* builds, and sometimes they suddenly do or say things that, in hindsight, they regret and say, 'Damn, what happened? I didn't mean to!' But it never happens without that tension.

For example, I think of a woman who came to therapy with her partner. She's a kindergarten teacher, patient and loving with the children—she has never lost her temper with them. That's a lot to manage. But in conflict with her husband, she can completely lose control. She doesn't understand the contrast: 'I'm normally a sweet, quiet woman. But when he acts cold and distant—like I'm talking to a wall—it drives me crazy! Then it's like I don't exist.' She tries everything to get a reaction, to feel seen. She told me that last week she smashed a vase on his head. He had a deep cut. On the way to the doctor, she was ashamed to tears and could hardly believe she had done that. This couple is experiencing violence. We can safely say that."

Welcome with the entire iceberg

Several new elements emerge when considering partner violence: it involves not only what couples themselves perceive as harmful and undesirable but also processes like tension-building. More pieces of the puzzle will follow, without reducing the entire dynamic to a single definition. The danger of a diagnostic or medicalized approach is that it isolates behavior from its context, a common pitfall in both society and the media. What follows is an effort to visualize that context and situate behavior within it.

Jef: "Partner violence, whether physical, verbal, social, sexual, or economic, occurs within a context. When you remove that context, it becomes dangerous. Think of the story of a ship that sank because people were looking only for icebergs above the water. They were scanning for white dots and chunks on the surface, forgetting that the largest part was hidden below. Of course, the actual story is more nuanced, but the point stands: we often only see the tip of the iceberg. You can't separate the visible from the invisible. The danger is in zooming in only on what's above the surface. The bulk—what lies beneath—is often invisible. That's the context. In this book, we want to focus on the whole iceberg. Partner violence isn't just about what's visible. That visible part is real, and we must acknowledge it—we cannot, should not, and will not ignore it. But we also have to consider everything happening beneath the surface that contributes to what eventually becomes visible. There is a societal tendency to focus solely on the violent acts. Everyone steers their boat while watching only the tops of icebergs: 'Watch out! That's where the danger is!' Meanwhile, the massive part below the surface is largely ignored. We want to honor that complexity. To people caught in cycles of escalation, we say: if you're confronting the tip of an iceberg in your relationship, welcome the entire iceberg, both the visible and the hidden parts. Because when partner violence surfaces, it's about more than just violence. It involves crucial issues like escalation, the loss of love, and disrupted attachment."

The context of society

Whenever one side of a duality is emphasized, the need arises to make the other side visible. It's unfortunate that two people and their relationship are so often reduced to the violence occurring between them. Yet, when the pain of that violence is denied space, something resists. In doing so, we also fail those individuals and their relationship. Perhaps that's why it takes two people to have this conversation—just as it takes two people to form a relationship dynamic. Lieven again shifts focus to the visible behavior: violence.

Lieven: "What's beneath the surface is crucial—and we'll spend a lot of time discussing that—but we also can't turn away from what happens above the waterline. Sometimes things spiral out of control—there can even be physical aggression. Society and the law are becoming increasingly clear: you cannot physically harm your partner. This is called violence, and society draws a firm line—this is not permitted. That's not up to us; it's something society defines. For example, we're one of the last countries in Western Europe where corporal punishment is still allowed in child-rearing. In Sweden, it's been illegal since 1976. Chances are that corporal punishment will eventually be banned here too. A hundred years ago, it was simply called 'discipline.' When things get out of hand in a relationship, couples often realize they don't want this, but society also increasingly sees it as unacceptable. The broader message is: '*Be careful*. This can cause lasting harm.'"

The first response to the question, "Is this partner violence?" should be: "Be careful—this question isn't risk-free when applied to relationship dynamics." Second, we observe that overly strict definitions can detach us from the broader context and obscure a more process-oriented inquiry: *What is happening within, between, and around people that leads to violence?* This is how we aim to do justice to the entire iceberg. Another layer of context then becomes visible: what we define today as partner violence—in a given society, at a given time—is not necessarily what was considered violence 50 years ago. Whether something qualifies as violence can depend on when and where you live. That, too, is context.

Crossing the line

Above the waterline, we encounter a societal perspective shaped by the spirit of the time and place in which one lives—this is where behaviors are judged as partner violence or not. Definitions of partner violence typically reside above the waterline. It's also the realm where actions occur that neither partner wants, as they harm both individuals and the relationship. This space can be described as the moment when something shifts. What begins as relational tension escalates, spiraling out of control and placing the couple in a situation neither intended. Partner violence becomes most visible above the waterline, even though a buildup often precedes it.

Jef: "We've spoken with countless people whose relationships spiraled out of control, where one or both partners reacted aggressively. Almost all of them say, 'I didn't want that!' And yet, it happens. And it causes suffering. Like the woman from the couple I mentioned earlier—during an argument, she hears herself saying her husband is worthless and that he shows no commitment to her or their daughter. In her rage, she tears down the father in him because she wants him to feel some of the pain she is feeling at that moment. Later, she tells me how much it hurts her to say that because his role as a father is what she loves most about him. Yet with one outburst, she obliterates that. She sees how it makes him question himself as a father and how it diminishes his involvement with their children. It's the last thing she wants to do. Just like, at one point, he slaps his wife so hard that the imprint of his hand remains on her face. That's not the man he wants to be. And yet, this is what happens between them.

I don't want to make the visible part of partner violence invisible. What I mean is that something shifts in a conversation when we fail to acknowledge the underlying dynamics, and simply say, 'That's violence. That's not allowed.' When we do that, neither the man nor the woman can say, 'I don't think this is okay,' because nearly everyone says that on their own—if given the space to do so. When they don't get that space, and we rush to judgment, they feel judged. And that doesn't help. It shuts a door. If there's one thing my work with couples dealing with violence has taught me, it's this: there is almost always something present that people feel ashamed of and afraid to talk about. That *shame* only grows under judgment. After all, we live in a world where partner violence is taboo and rarely met with compassion."

Lieven: "I keep saying that part of this is justified, Jef. That's how society signals: we do not accept this. Shame comes with that because society condemns it. That's how a community communicates to its members: don't do this, it causes harm. And many people already carry that shame within them. They don't necessarily need society to tell them—it's already felt. We know that most people who have responded physically in a relationship feel that inner shame. They think, 'I didn't really want that.' But that's not true for everyone. I emphasize this perspective because there are also readers who will say, 'I wasn't the one who got violent—I was the one who got hit.' We need to welcome them too. Some will say, 'That was partner violence,' to clarify something for their partner, to say, 'I don't want this. This crossed a line.' They are searching for a way to make that boundary clear, and they don't always feel strong enough to do it alone. Society helps them voice that line."

Jef: "Absolutely. Welcome to the readers who have experienced something in their relationship that felt unacceptable. To express that clearly to a partner, they may need society, a therapist, other people—or a definition—to help communicate that a line was crossed. In essence, they're saying, 'I don't want things in our relationship to spiral so far out of control.' In that sense, I welcome them as people fighting for their relationships—as relationship improvers. To better understand this shift in thinking, we return to the iceberg metaphor. The question, 'Is this partner violence?' directs us to the tip of the iceberg. But if we want to understand the relational meaning behind the question, we must look below the surface—to the submerged, often invisible part of the iceberg. That's what the next chapter is about."

The subjectivity of partners

We return to the heart of the original question: *Is this partner violence?* Subjectivity is essential in answering this. It's important to acknowledge the complexity of escalating conflict, while also recognizing a simple truth: if someone experiences something as violent, then for them, it is. In that moment, something harmful is happening. Their perception matters—and we must take it seriously. From this perspective, people seeking an answer don't need a definition. What matters is their lived experience. As a couple, they must work with that reality. To those individuals, we say: *Welcome to the pain you're experiencing in this relationship that means so much to you.* Because that's what their subjective reality communicates. Subjectivity is a critical piece in the puzzle of partner violence. But so is the term itself—*partner violence*—which holds another key component.

Lieven: "We're talking about violence—more specifically, *partner* violence. That word includes *partner*, and that part is indispensable. If you are single, you cannot speak of partner violence. It is something that occurs within a relationship between two people who have entered into a meaningful, often positive, alliance. This distinguishes it from other forms of violence, such as street violence, which, as the name suggests, occurs in public, or hooligan violence, which might break out after a soccer game. Partner violence is not just violence in general. The term itself brings in a specific context: the intimate relationship. It is violence that takes place within a particular setting. And it's precisely the nature of this setting—the interactional dynamics, the emotional closeness, the unique features of a couple as a small system—that creates conditions for both deeply meaningful and enjoyable experiences *and* the potential for things to spiral out of control. In the next two chapters, we will explore how and why such escalation can happen specifically within the context of a romantic partnership. That's not a coincidence. It has everything to do with the nature of the relationship and its particular characteristics."

Partner and violence: Two parts, one word. We explore the danger of separating "partner" and "violence"—of turning a single word into two. When we isolate violence from the relationship, failing to recognize the human, loving context in which it occurs, we risk losing something essential. This detachment is dangerous because it obscures critical dynamics, and in response, people may escalate conflict in an attempt to make themselves seen. Conversely, it's equally problematic to focus solely on the partnership and the relationship—responding only with empathy and understanding. We must not minimize the violence or overlook the harm it causes. There has to be something in us, and around us, that firmly says: "This can't and shouldn't happen." That voice exists both within society and within individuals who struggle with partner violence. It's already present in the reader because everyone feels this tension.

But when the environment only points a finger and shouts, "Not allowed! Unacceptable! Over the line!" we risk pushing people into polarized positions. They stop hearing each other—let alone understanding each other. In such a polarized atmosphere, how can they possibly find their way back to one another?

It makes more sense to hold the two parts of the word—partner and violence—together. When we do, we can acknowledge both the violence and the submerged iceberg beneath the surface: the contextual buildup in which something occurs that neither the partners nor society find acceptable. It is this often invisible buildup that we want to bring into the light—something society rarely welcomes.

Intimate terrorism versus situational couple violence

To better understand partner violence and its associated dynamics, it is crucial to make an important distinction. The literature differentiates between *intimate terrorism* (or coercive controlling violence) and *situational couple violence*. As stated in the introduction, this book focuses on the latter. We are not addressing instrumental violence or coercive control, but rather a loving relationship in which interactions spiral out of control at certain moments. This distinction is difficult to make, because behaviorally, on the surface, these situations can look quite similar. But below the surface, the dynamics are very different.

Jef: "The type of partner violence we're talking about occurs within a relational dynamic in which violence—verbal, physical, sexual, social, financial—is the visible tip of the iceberg. It still takes place within a context of love and assumed equality. That's different from a relationship where one person systematically uses the other. There's an underwater dynamic there too, but it's fundamentally different. Unfortunately, these two forms are often confused, especially in public discourse. We sometimes use simpler terms: hot and cold partner violence. In 'hot' violence, emotions, warmth, and love are still present between partners. In 'cold' violence, there's no love—not even hidden or disguised. It's stripped of humanity. This cold form *is actually rare*, though it's often the first image people associate with partner violence."

Lieven: "In a healthy partner relationship, you contribute to something greater than yourself. Of course, you do things for each other, but it doesn't feel like being used. It's mutual. If you start keeping score—'I've done more than you'—that's a red flag for the relationship's future. A healthy relationship rests on mutual investment in the shared good. Yes, you may sometimes feel you've given too much, but that alone doesn't make the relationship cold. Coldness emerges when giving becomes a pattern of strategic self-interest—when one partner no longer considers the other's inner world. That's when we may be dealing with abuse."

Jef: "What exactly constitutes cold versus hot violence is difficult to convey because, on the surface, we often observe the same behaviors and sometimes even the same words. We have studied literature and research on partner violence for years. Together, we have spoken to hundreds of couples experiencing this issue and have provided training worldwide on the topic. When people ask, 'Is this cold? Is this abuse?' one thing we have learned is that, in the vast majority of cases, it is not intimate terrorism but situational couple violence. Cold abuse accounts for only a very small percentage.

Moreover, when people ask how to understand their relationship dynamics so they can change their behavior, there is a strong likelihood that they are dealing with the hot form—situational partner violence. In cases of intimate terrorism, this question typically does not apply to both partners. Those involved *rarely seek help voluntarily* as a couple. To clearly explain the difference between situational partner violence and intimate terrorism—or hot versus cold violence—we actually need to discuss love, the loss of love, and attachment. This topic is addressed in question 2. Trying to distinguish between the two without understanding these underlying dynamics leaves you stuck—you may notice this in our discussion now. Hot partner violence has an underlying dynamic beneath the surface, which can be understood through attachment, mutuality, and (the loss of) love. Cold violence, abuse, or intimate terrorism lacks that dynamic. It is a *one-way*, instrumental form of violence."

Lieven: "We realize we are challenging readers here and may leave them wanting a clearer explanation of intimate terrorism. In the next chapter (question 2), we explore situational partner violence in depth. The general tendency is to first ask, 'What is cold?' but we choose not to start there. Instead, we begin by examining the connection between the relationship context and violence. Then we

> explore the underlying dynamics, allowing the distinction between hot and cold to emerge naturally. If the warm, underlying dynamic is absent, the violence might be cold.
>
> We believe it is essential to make this connection, and we deliberately choose to start by searching for heat. That is a conscious choice because if you focus on looking for cold, you will find it—even when the situation is actually warm."

We choose to focus on the warm dynamics. This choice is grounded both in our years of experience and in scientific research. The distinction between intimate terrorism and situational partner violence frequently appears in the literature. What this consistently shows is that the warm form—situational partner violence—is by far the most common. Overall, 24.6% of people have asked themselves the question, "What's going on between us? Is this partner violence?" Within that group, the vast majority involves situational partner violence. Research always attempts to portray reality, though it rarely captures all the nuances, especially when studying partner violence. For example, different studies use varying criteria to define intimate terrorism: some emphasize the severity and frequency of violence, while others focus more on motive (power). It is also notable that research predominantly addresses male violence, while female violence is rarely considered in the data. Bearing these limitations in mind, we still provide some illustrative findings. For instance, one study (Dutton & Nichols, 2005) showed that only 1 in 200 men arrested for partner violence were involved in intimate terrorism. Another statistic indicates that only 3% of male violence cases involve repeated serious violence (Straus & Gelles, 1992). These are among the more reliable studies and convey a key message: although the general perspective and approach to partner violence focus almost exclusively on intimate terrorism, experiences of conflicts that truly escalate overwhelmingly arise from situational partner violence dynamics. Moreover, in nearly 60% of these cases, violence is bi-directional—emanating from both partners simultaneously.

Conclusion: a nuanced story

Although we were initially hesitant to define when partner violence occurs, we ultimately incorporated many elements that get to the core of escalating conflict. These are boundary-crossing experiences in a relationship where one or both partners feel, "This is going too far; I don't want this. This is not us." Perception is crucial here. The external behaviors visible during these conflicts may include verbal, sexual, physical, social, or economic expressions. Equally important is the less visible internal aspect: the buildup within the interactions and the inner worlds of both partners involved. While discussions about partner violence often divide couples into perpetrators and victims, literature and research show that, in the vast majority of cases, the reality is far more nuanced.

We began with the question, "Is it partner violence?" This evolved into, "What form of partner violence is it?" To that, we can answer: "Most likely, it is situational violence paradoxically connected to love." How these two seemingly contradictory concepts relate leads to the next common and logical question couples ask: "Do we love each other when we hurt each other so much?" The underlying dynamics of this situational form of partner violence in the majority of cases are explored in the next chapter.

Reflect and relate

Take a moment to pause and connect these ideas to your own experience.

The questions below are not meant to judge or define your relationship. They are an invitation to reflect on what happens between you and your partner—and within yourself—when conflicts arise, lines are crossed, or love feels out of reach.

1. Have you ever felt, in your current or a previous relationship: "This feels like intimate partner violence"?

2. Do you recognize the feeling in such moments: "This isn't what I want. This crosses a line. This isn't who we are"?

3. Imagine telling a close friend, "That moment… it crossed a line for me. That's not who we are as a couple."

4. How would it feel to say that out loud?

5. If you were to ask your partner in a calm moment, "Did you also feel that things got out of hand—that it didn't fit with who we are?" What do you think he or she would say?

6. In this chapter, we differentiated between two forms of violence in relationships—one rooted in escalating conflict and the other in control and domination. Although this distinction is meaningful, it can be difficult to make in the heat of conflict or escalation.

7. If you recognize that love is still present between you and your partner, and that your conflicts seem to have a relational buildup, we want to encourage you to continue reading this book.

References

Dutton, D. G., & Nichols, T. L. (2005). The gender paradigm in domestic violence research and theory: Part 1-the conflict of theory and data. *Aggression and Violent Behavior*, 10, 680–714.

Straus, M. A., & Gelles, R. J. (1992). How violent are American families? In M. A. Straus, & R. J. Gelles (Eds.), *Physical violence in American families* (pp. 95–108). Transaction Publishers.

2
DO WE LOVE EACH OTHER WHEN WE HURT EACH OTHER SO MUCH?

People who love each other do not want to hurt one another. Those we love, we want to protect, cherish, help grow, and see enjoy life. We wish for our loved ones everything except misfortune, pain, sorrow, and suffering. Yet, it happens all over the world. No one escapes from it. Pain seems inherent in love. Anyone who connects with someone and shares love will also encounter pain. In itself, there is nothing wrong with that. No day without night. No love without pain. In many couples, however, these conflicts escalate. What begins as a misunderstanding, a disagreement, or slight tension can deteriorate into repeated, sharp words that sear into the soul and cannot be erased. Sometimes it is not only words that deliver blows; sometimes the blows are literal—a push that ends with a nasty fall, a punch that leaves a black eye, nails that scratch open an entire back. These wounds also heal with difficulty. When a couple experiences this, their love is often questioned. Once they have recovered from the blow, they are frequently left wondering whether they really love each other when they can hurt each other so much. Can love cause so much damage?

Before addressing this question, we need to revisit the distinction between two forms of partner violence: situational partner violence (hot) and intimate terrorism (cold). These forms are driven by different dynamics. In hot

DOI: 10.4324/9781003683582-3

violence—the form from which the vast majority of couples experiencing partner violence suffer—violence and love are two sides of the same coin. Cold violence, or intimate terrorism, however, has nothing to do with love. This, of course, raises the question: Is it hot or cold with us? If you recognize what we describe in the following chapter, assume it is the hot form.

The illusion of painless love

It is entirely natural for people to wonder whether love can still exist when they hurt, scratch, bite, and shout the sharpest, most hurtful, reproachful things at each other. This is deeply confusing, so of course people ask themselves that question. The violence frightens and overwhelms. It makes it even harder to feel the partner's love—yet love, especially the threat of losing it, is the core of the dynamic they are caught in. To understand this dangerous but loving dynamic, we must begin at the beginning: the start of a relationship. At this point, two issues emerge that sow the seeds for the severe escalations that may follow.

Lieven: "When we start a romantic relationship and someone likes us, we feel something like, 'Finally! Someone who loves me.' If all goes well, that is a wonderful experience. 'Life is beautiful! I didn't know it could be so beautiful.' It gives you a kind of hope that all good things will come your way. Even if you had a good time before, you suddenly feel much better. Everything is possible; life smiles at you. At the beginning of a relationship, we all enter that dream to some extent. It makes you think it is impossible for violence to occur in something so beautiful. Although, even at the start, there can be robust bickering or tension as both partners try to find their place in the relationship. Even though those awkward moments exist, the intensity of the positive moments makes us forget them. In that context, the thought arises: *if you love each other, there can be no pain.* That is the first illusion often held by fledgling relationships.

A second, essential element is this: *no one can hurt you as much as the one you love.* That makes it logical that we react so strongly when your partner doesn't understand you or believes something about you that you don't think is true. When your loved one makes a joke and you don't laugh... that already hurts... let alone when it concerns important matters. Yesterday, in a training session, I spoke about a couple. The man in that relationship often wanted to make love. The woman no longer felt like it. When we explored this further, it became clear that the man's pain was this: 'I want to show you so much that I love you, and every time I try, you see me as a dirty sex maniac. It hurts so much that you don't see me the way I see myself. That you don't see my love.' It's about things like that."

"Finally!", a romantic ideal

A relationship often begins with the illusion that hurting is not part of love. In reality, pain is part of love—simply because no one else's opinion or view matters as much. No one can hurt us as deeply as the person who lives in our heart. Reflecting on this illusion naturally leads us to the work of Justine van Lawick, a Dutch psychologist and teacher, specializing in fighting divorces and violence in families. Alongside Martine Groen, she did invaluable work in the Netherlands, making violence in relationships a topic that could be openly discussed and creating space to work with couples on this complex issue. Both women deserve much credit. What Justine and Martine articulate so clearly—and which aligns closely with the illusion just described—is that people experiencing violence in relationships often begin from a 'romantic ideal.' This concept captures the imagination. Jef explains:

Jef: "People meet, and somehow that meeting feels magical. When you ask couples about the beginning—about their first encounters—they often describe an experience like this: 'Finally, someone who sees who I am. Finally, someone who sees what I do and can do. Finally, someone who understands me. Finally, someone who comforts me. Finally, someone with whom I can have fun and feel free. Finally, someone with whom I can be myself and be loved for who I am.' Yesterday, I spoke with a couple who suffer greatly from violence, and they put it like this: 'Finally, someone who doesn't denigrate me. Finally, someone with whom I can feel equality.' The key word in all those statements is Finally! Somehow, that word feels healing. I think that's why Justine van Lawick speaks of the 'romantic ideal from the traumatic connection.' Trauma sounds heavy, but it doesn't always have to be. The experience is valid even without trauma. No one grows up without heartache or rejection. We have all been small and vulnerable while growing up, and we have all been scratched in the process. We have all experienced enough pain to feel 'Finally!' Of course, some wounds are deeper, larger, and more painful, which makes the 'Finally!' even more intense—insane, in the sense of, 'I didn't know this existed!' In that way, it's a spectrum. The more you have missed in life, the more magnetic and enchanting something nurturing becomes. If you've missed a lot of love, security, or warmth and suddenly experience that long-awaited love or warmth… that's fantastic."

Love works like a magnet. The feeling of 'Finally!' causes something to click between two people, and that is wonderful. However, magnets also have the property that if you flip them, they no longer attract—they repel. This is the other side of the story: no one can hurt you like the one you love so deeply—the one who makes you feel that intense 'Finally!' Suddenly, the magnetic force reverses, and very painful things happen.

The greater the loss, the louder the 'Finally!' and the bigger the disillusionment that arises from cracks appearing in that 'Finally!' It will hurt at some point, but the intensity of losing the 'Finally!' grows as the underlying pain and absence deepen. The 'Finally!' says, 'The pain is over,' but in reality, the pain remains in your body—it doesn't disappear. As Alfons Vansteenwegen—a well-known Flemish sexologist and couples therapist—puts it: after the dream phase, reality arrives, and with reality comes difference. That inevitably means your partner will fail you at some point. This reopens the pain beneath. To truly understand that pain, we need to address the attachment questions underneath.

Lieven: "You meet someone, you fall in love, and you feel how wonderful that is. The 'Finally!' you feel at that moment is relief after vulnerability. At its core, the 'Finally!' answers two or three questions: *'Am I good enough for you?'*—'Whew, finally, I'm more than good enough just being myself!' or *'Are you there for me?'*—'Whew, finally, there's someone who really wants to be there for me!' You can add, *'Do I belong?'*—'Whew, I'm finally coming home and becoming part of something.' These are three key questions in adult love relationships to understand the 'Finally!' That's what attachment theory and Sue Johnson taught us. She is a Canadian psychologist, researcher, professor, the founder of EFT, and a world-renowned author of several books on relationship therapy who translated this complex issue into human words. If we put it simply, it becomes: 'Finally, there is someone for me! Finally, I am good enough in someone's eyes! Finally, I belong somewhere.' Or still: 'I'm seen, just as I am.' Sometimes you were only seen when you were breaking things or being awkward. Sometimes you were only seen if you worked hard enough or performed perfectly. Now, you are seen without having to try. And that is wonderful. It is the desire of every human being to be seen for who they are, without having to do or be anything else."

A crack in the ice

Jef: "If we experience the feeling of 'Finally!' for a while, love begins to arise. If that feeling lasts longer, a deeper love emerges—a love rooted in 'I am good enough, I matter, I am seen, I come home...' But when we let people into our hearts, we take a risk. You let them in, allow them to get closer, and then you dare to show yourself more than usual. Very concretely: you start to dare to take off your clothes.

You reveal yourself naked. Sexuality symbolizes what happens in a relationship. You allow yourself to be touched; you show your vulnerabilities. In that moment, love and the feeling of connection grow—and alongside it, the risk you take grows too. When I expose myself so vulnerably, and then there is a little laughter... that hurts deeply. In the outside world, with people where I don't feel that 'Finally!' connection, I can handle it because there I'm not naked. But here, I am unprotected. If my partner does something that gives me the impression, 'You don't like me. I'm not okay for you. I don't belong anymore...' a rupture appears in the 'Finally!'

I picture you standing on a very solid piece of concrete—or a thick sheet of ice, to use the metaphor of Jim Furrow, an American theologian, relationship and family therapist, researcher, and EFT trainer. You two stand on the ice. It is thick, you feel stability and firmness. From this place, you can handle the world. Suddenly, something happens between you. Your partner says something that really hurts you, and... crack. A crack in the ice, in the platform on which you stand together. Panic! This is frightening. It's precisely because we have a safe connection and safe love—because we experience the 'Finally!'—and then inevitably lose it again, that this moment can become a starting point. People begin fighting for love. In that context, it's not unusual to hurt each other when you love each other."

Lieven: "That sense of nakedness is so recognizable—the physical, but especially the psychological nakedness. We all know it. You meet someone you really like, and suddenly you share things you have never told anyone before. That is very intimate and special. When insecurity enters that nakedness, it can be very intense. Suddenly, her friends arrive, and she laughs at something revealing about him—or suddenly, her own vulnerability about a difficult relationship with her parents erupts as 'You're just like your mother!' Then, clearly, this can be very painful.

The bottom line is that the 'Finally!' inevitably gets broken at some point. There is no avoiding it. This is the story of all couples; it is not limited to those suffering from violence. When that magic breaks, *fear* enters. How couples deal with that fear makes all the difference. Research shows that violence is most common among young couples—adolescents and young students. That has a lot to do with brain development. The frontal lobes aren't fully developed yet, so perspective-taking is more difficult. It also relates to the intensity of emotions at that age. When the 'Finally!' breaks in this context, it can quickly escalate into violence. Those couples break up more often, I suspect.

When couples stay together longer, they experience the 'Finally!', the rupture in it that awakens fear, and a certain interaction cycle rooted in that fear. As they grow through this process, they can rebuild a kind of 'Finally!', but of a different nature—more nuanced and enduring. It is a process over time. Time is important. You can think of the repeated experiences of 'Finally!' as bricks drying in the sun. If you have shared many 'Finally!' moments, those become solid bricks you can use to build a stable, strong home. Then the house—the home—becomes more important and durable than the intense but brief feeling of 'Finally!' In that home, you know love can also hurt, but that is not threatening because you understand the home can be shaken and repaired. You know that a little damage does not mean the house will collapse: there is trust that, together, you will fix it."

The evolution of protection

The magnetic attraction of the initial feeling of coming home to someone—finally being understood and truly allowed to be yourself for the first time—is inevitably broken. This naturally generates anxiety, which we manage by stepping into certain interaction patterns. These patterns serve as protection against the unpredictability of losing the 'Finally!' feeling. While they may work well in the short term, in the long run, they often lead to more escalations. Couples can begin to work through this partly by understanding each other's protective responses. To reach that understanding, it helps first to recognize how this protection is evolutionarily rooted.

Jef: "To understand how fear can spill over into conflict, it's important to consider how we are naturally equipped to protect ourselves from losing a sense of home. This traces back to the fact that we are herd animals—mammals, tribal beings. To survive, we evolved to relate and connect. Sue Johnson has suggested that 'homo empathicus' would be a better name for us because humans possess a system focused on sensing how everyone around us is feeling. We can make deep connections with one another, and we do this for a reason: it was essential for survival millions of years ago. We needed—and still need—a tribe to survive. We cannot do it alone.

What happens when you are threatened within the tribe? The tribe's function is to protect against outside threats, but sometimes the threat arises from within. There may be a quarrel, you feel exposed in your nakedness, and then... we are naturally equipped to protect ourselves from the overwhelming fear of losing the tribe, our relationships, our home—because that would be life-threatening for our species. Today, the tribe is primarily a partner relationship. There is a lot of pressure on this relationship. In the past, you had the village or community; now it is the small family, with the partner as a key foundation. Readers may be familiar with the system nature gave us when danger is imminent: fight or flight. When something threatens the loss of our tribe, we raise our voices and protest: 'I live with you in a home I don't want to lose. I refuse to lose you! You hurt me, and I protest!' That is the fight mode. There has been a breach in the solid foundation we stood on, and I fight to protect it. This is a strategy we knew as babies. A baby who loses contact after birth cries out, 'Where are you?!' They are reassured when placed on a body, feeling a heartbeat and contact. Here we see how innate this tendency is. Consider, for example, little monkeys who, when danger threatens, cling to their mother's fur. Many people do the same, figuratively—they 'cling.' That is one protective strategy. The other is flight: to 'weather the storm' by getting quiet and waiting it out. If I keep moving forward without fully feeling the fear, it will pass. In English, this is called 'to turtle'—pulling your head into your shell. In Flemish, we say 'Head in sand!'—don't feel too much, bow down, and survive."

Lieven: "We are attachment thinkers, right, Jef? So we can replace the tribe with the idea of 'home.' Coming home means entering a tribe where you are good enough and seen—where you belong. Within your home, you feel protected from the rest of the world. If something threatening happens within that home, you'll either 'turtle' or 'hold tight.' There is nothing wrong with either response. Both are necessary. If you never raise your voice, it's important to learn to stand up for yourself. And if you always want everything immediately, it's important to learn to wait. We have been practicing this since children were two years old: 'Wait a minute. Not right away.' Being able to wait and to speak up are both positive skills. If this works well, the other person hears you, fear subsides, and calm returns. So it depends on the response—it is crucial. If a baby cries and the parents respond by showing up, the baby's needs are met. If a four-year-old sits at the table and the parents say, 'Wait a minute, mommy and daddy are speaking, but soon it will be your turn,' and the child waits and then is heard—well done. It is hard for a four-year-old to wait because they want to be listened to, but they learn to trust that the other person will listen and that they are allowed to be there. Here's the point: if repeated experiences teach us that waiting is followed by being heard, that sometimes we need to speak louder to be noticed but then are effectively heard, safety arises. A stable sense develops: I have a solid house where I am okay in the eyes of others; I have ways to be seen and to feel that I am good enough. The shakier the house, with bigger cracks in the foundation, the less effective 'turtling' or 'holding tight' becomes—and the greater the panic grows. Then we start shouting louder or remaining silent for longer periods. We carry the experience of needing to shout very loudly or stay very quiet into the next home."

Pursuing and withdrawing in action

When we love, we risk loss. That loss is inevitable: the loss of a long-awaited connection, the loss of a home, or the loss of a sense of belonging. Our brains are naturally equipped with strategies to defend against such loss. Two fundamental responses are hardwired into us: protest ("Hold on tightly") and withdrawal ("Turtling"). In attachment theory, these are known as *pursuing* and *withdrawing*. Let's take a closer look.

Jef: "It reminds me of Franco and Anna. They went out together and had a great evening—dinner with friends, dancing, laughter, a few drinks, and lots of conversation. When they wake up the next morning, they still feel the magic of the night before, but they're also tired and slightly hungover.

As Franco wakes, he thinks, *We'll get up, and then we'll have two hours before we need to pick up the kids from Grandma's. We could take that time for a nice, relaxed breakfast together... hold on to that feeling from yesterday.* He's having a harder time getting out of bed than Anna, who is already downstairs.

She walks into the living room and immediately notices the mess: *Oh no, that coat's on the floor. The shoes are on the sofa. He had another drink and left everything behind. A glass has toppled over on the table, and the leftover whiskey has spilled and dried into a sticky mess on the table and floor.*

Damn, she thinks. *I still have to clean all this up—and I want it done before we head to my parents' house.*

Meanwhile, Franco is still caught in the warmth of yesterday's mood as he comes downstairs. But when he sees Anna, he senses something is off.

Uh-oh, he thinks. *She seems angry. What did I do wrong?* This is where the conversation begins.

'Honey, everything okay?' he asks gently, trying to check in.

'Yes, everything is just fine,' Anna replies flatly. He moves to give her a hug, but she pulls back.

'Just let me clean this,' she says.

Franco backs off and sits down at the table. 'Okay.'

To which Anna responds, with a hint of sarcasm, 'You really don't have to help, you know.'

A deep sigh from Franco. A raised eyebrow from Anna.

Here, a familiar pattern of interaction begins to emerge—one that many couples will recognize. It can be summed up as the classic 'What's wrong?—Nothing!' dynamic. When one partner feels blocked in their attempt to reconnect, they begin to wonder what's going on. *What happened? Why can't I feel you anymore?* That uncertainty is often expressed as the question: *What's wrong?*

But the partner on the receiving end of that question may not hear it as, *I miss you; I'm scared we've lost something.* Instead, it often lands as: *Am I doing something wrong? Am I not okay as I am? Is my burden unwelcome?* It's no surprise, then, that the response is often defensive, either through sharp words or through a sharp silence. A loud, clipped *Nothing!* or a cold, distant one.

Do you feel the tension building?

Let that tension linger unresolved for a while, and conflict—a discussion, an argument, or even an escalation—won't be far behind."

From protecting to fighting

Lieven: "Well… I know that story. I know it all too well myself, and I've heard many people share it. What's more, when someone responds with 'Nothing,' it's rarely said with a smile or a calm, reassuring expression. The face says, *Something serious is going on!* The connection that the partner desperately needs in that moment doesn't happen. To return to our metaphor: the house they built together is still standing, but it's starting to wobble. The vagueness and fear felt by one partner lead them either to insist or to withdraw in silence. We can all imagine how that unfolds. Phrases like, 'If you keep saying nothing is wrong, then there will be something!' often arise. At that point, two innate tendencies come into play. The question, 'Everything okay?!' has an impact on the sense of security within the house. If one partner senses tension, so does the other. Every couple, everywhere in the world, encounters this at some point. These behaviors in themselves are not the problem—on the contrary. They are natural protective responses. Speaking clearly is an attempt to reestablish contact. Silence is an attempt to preserve connection, not to sever it. Sometimes, this works well. But for many couples, this dynamic solidifies into a pattern. Over time, it can become rigid, and the escalations intensify. The louder the silence, the louder the speaking. These reactions can reinforce each other."

Jef: "This is the point where powerlessness spills over into physical wordlessness. It begins with something seemingly small: the facial expression. A sigh, a raised eyebrow, a furrowed brow, an averted gaze, a tight mouth… But over time, the pattern can become so ingrained that it manifests more strongly: a sharp tone of voice, darting eyes, turning away, walking out of the room—and in some cases, even physical harm. The body always speaks. So this conflict always reveals itself through the body."

In the first stage—meeting and falling in love—there inevitably comes a moment of loss: the end of the *Finally!* feeling. In the second stage—when the relationship expands and deepens into love—there is sometimes a sense of losing your home. A crack appears in the sense of safety. The vulnerability of emotional nakedness can turn something that's merely frightening into something threatening. And what threatens one partner inevitably threatens the other, because it happens within their shared home. Suddenly, the home feels unstable. Each person reacts from a place of protection, either with fearful silence or with defensive anger, both of which make the home feel even more unsteady. That's when protection can start to turn into aggression.

Sue Johnson once said in her North American way, "We cracked the code of love," which may sound grandiose. But with this kind of understanding and the underlying lens of attachment, we gain a way to decode the complex dynamics of a couple and truly listen to what's going on. The same love that comforts us in places where we've been wounded is the love that can also hurt us or scare us. Love and fear are deeply intertwined. We are vulnerable in this house we are building together—precisely because it matters so much. The loss of safety in your shared home is so threatening because it can lead to the loss of the home itself. And then you are exposed—not only to each other but also to the world. That is profoundly unsettling.

Lieven: "When we've finally found and built a home, we naturally fear losing it. When the other person goes out with friends and comes back later than expected, treats the children differently than you would like, or doesn't seem as gentle as in the beginning… it creates doubt. At first, you might think: 'Wow, what a tidy man!' Later that might become: 'Wow, he's so rigid.' Or: 'What a delightfully zany, funny person,' might shift to: 'Can he never be serious?' You may have thought: 'Such a caring woman,' and later feel: 'She always has to know everything about me.' Or even: 'She's so full of life!' only to find yourself thinking: 'Morning thunderstorm, afternoon sunshine, evening hurricane… I'm exhausted. I can't keep up.' Or you thought, 'Finally, someone brings predictability into my life!' and eventually, 'This feels like control. I didn't ask for that, did I?' These are the moments when something beautiful starts to show its cracks."

Jef: "You've described very precisely the moment when something frightening starts to creep into that *Finally!* which, over time, has become a home. That's when fear enters. And when we're afraid, we often become threatening to the person we love. At that point, our innate attachment strategies kick in—we start defending ourselves against the fear of losing our home and our love.

We'll go into the different interaction patterns that result from this in the next chapter. For now, let's summarize: the house develops a crack. We get scared. In a desperate search for reassurance, we engage in behaviors that are meant to protect us, but that the other person experiences as threatening. And in response, they also protect themselves in ways that amplify the fear, rather than soothe it. Some couples manage to break out of this dynamic. These are the ones who, over time, find ways to reassure one another. But others don't. In those relationships, fear and a sense of threat gradually fill the home until the walls begin to buckle.

Couples who can reassure one another begin to realize: 'My self-protection hurts my partner.' For example: 'My harsh criticism hurts him—it makes him feel like I don't think he's good enough.' Or: 'My cold silence hurts her—it makes her feel like I don't want to be with her.' Recognizing and accepting that pain is crucial for breaking the cycle. But when things spiral out of control—because the conflicts are intense or repeated over time—the insecurity in the home doesn't go away, even during calm periods. The underlying pain is not understood, so it doesn't get resolved. Instead, it lingers like a toxic, invisible gas. Things may seem fine, but we're no longer certain. A persistent sense of stress remains. And stress, after all, is a form of anxiety."

Lieven: "Of course, the story can also start the other way around: one person senses that something is wrong, feels tension or insecurity in the house, and decides, 'I'm not going to say anything. I'll stay quiet to avoid conflict. I'm not doing anything.' But that person *is* doing something. The other partner comes home, feeling everything is fine, and suddenly senses the silence. They see an expression that's not quite a smile and feel, *What's going on here?*—and just like that, fear is awakened. The interaction begins. It can start with either partner.

Some people take a step back when they're afraid—they try to become invisible. Others take a step forward—they seek contact. The latter are the ones who say, 'We need to talk.' Half the people reading this will know the feeling that phrase evokes: heart racing, a light sweat breaking out… And that's not just an adult experience. We learned it as children. When Mom or Dad said, 'We need to talk,' it usually meant something was wrong. 'What happened at school?' or, 'We're getting a divorce,' or, 'Mom is sick,' or even, 'What did I find in your room? Is that cannabis?!' You get the picture. So even in adulthood, 'We need to talk,' can trigger a wave of anxiety—and ignite the entire couple dynamic."

Conclusion: from a warm house to hot violence

At the beginning of this book, we posed the question: *What is partner violence?* This naturally led us to distinguish between *hot* and *cold* aggression. We chose to focus on the heat—first, because it is by far the most common form, and, second, because if you go looking for cold aggression, you will inevitably find it. In any interaction pattern where violence occurs, cold elements are present. As a result, it becomes all too easy to conclude that we are dealing with cold aggression and cold people. But throughout the narrative we have laid out here, warmth is unmistakably present. We are telling a story that applies to all couples, but especially to those in which something deeply loving can, at times, turn into something violent and painful.

What we have described is the story of situational partner violence. We began with the experience of *Finally!*—that profound sense of arrival—and how that repeated feeling helps partners gather the building blocks for creating a home. This home is warm, offering protection and a sense of safety. It's a place that can withstand stress. Yet, insecurity can still find its way inside. That, in itself, is not unusual. Often, couples manage to regain control over that insecurity and push it out together. However, if that insecurity recurs too often or becomes too intense, it eventually saturates the emotional air the couple breathes. The house starts to feel unstable. Fear of losing it grows. People may become overwhelmed by helplessness. If this persists, they can find themselves trapped in escalating patterns of interaction—fierce and sometimes violent—as they try to protect themselves from the insecurity and the threat of losing their home. In that effort to defend, they may begin to hurt each other, both literally and emotionally. Thus, something born of warmth and love can give rise to behaviors so intense and painful that they seem cold. But beneath those dynamics, the warmth and the love still resonate.

The specific nature of these interaction patterns deserves careful attention. We will explore them in more detail in the next chapter. For now, we hope to have given you a sense of how loving connections can, over time, turn into cycles of pain—simply because love feels so good, and the fear of losing it feels so unsafe.

Reflect and relate

Take a moment to pause and connect these ideas to your own experience.

The questions below are not meant to judge or define your relationship. They are an invitation to reflect on what happens between you and your partner—and within yourself—when love, fear, and pain coexist.

1. Can you sense in what way your partner feels like your "finally"—how being in this relationship brings something precious that you have longed for in your life?

2. Can you recall moments when you lost touch with that "finally" feeling? How did your body tell you that something had changed? What went through your mind?

3. When this happens, how do you tend to move? Do you hold back and endure, or do you protest and reach out?

4. What impact does that movement have on the connection between you and your partner?

5. If you were to ask your partner what it looks like when they lose their "finally" feeling, what do you think they would say?

3
WHAT'S GOING ON BETWEEN US?!

"I yell something, he pushes me..."

"The more I say 'leave me alone!' the more she insists on talking about it... until suddenly we're shouting at each other and it gets physical."

"All I ask is for him to listen to me, but the more I insist, the more distant he becomes. At some point, he just walks away, and then I really freak out. I literally slam the door in his face. I mean... how cowardly can you be?"

Conflicts, especially those that escalate into violence, are deeply confusing and complicated. At the same time, they often seem to follow the same pattern. What are these dynamics that lead to violence? How can we make sense of what happens between partners when they fight? And how is it possible that such intense events can become predictable? Every couple experiences conflict, and every couple argues according to a certain pattern. This is no different for couples where violence occurs. In fact, the interactional patterns we see in violent relationships are not fundamentally different from those in nonviolent ones. They are simply much more intense.

DOI: 10.4324/9781003683582-4

In 2017—when we were trying to conceptualize our experiences with partner violence—we created a slide for a workshop titled: "Partner violence = ordinary conflict × 10." In this chapter, we will elaborate on the reasoning and structure behind that slide.

We will explain the relational dynamics that emerge when people feel disconnected from one another. Then, we will explore how this disconnection can escalate into violent intensity.

To be clear, we are talking specifically about *situational partner violence*. We are not addressing *intimate terrorism*, or what is sometimes referred to as the "cold" form of violence, which follows a very different dynamic.

The extraordinary—from within and without

As we explained in the previous chapter, many people are lucky enough to fall in love, find a home in another person, and feel deeply cared for. But life continually disrupts that ideal of finally being understood. If only because, as humans, we are not particularly skilled at understanding each other. We may listen, but that doesn't mean we truly hear one another. Sometimes, someone says something unusual—something extraordinary—and that disrupts the ordinary. That disruption is often the first element in the buildup of conflict.

Lieven: "This morning I spoke with Dirk and Nadia, a couple for whom 'togetherness' feels natural to Nadia. Doing things together is familiar to her—she grew up with it. Her parents did things as a unit. Not everything, but enough to make togetherness feel normal. Her background values the group over the individual. Like in soccer: the team is more important than the individual players. Dirk, however, comes from a very different world. He was neglected as a child. His parents were rarely present, and when they were, there was little emotional connection. They didn't do much as a couple. According to Dirk, his mother constantly criticized his father, who took it silently. The children were sent to boarding school. So, when Nadia suggests doing something together, it's an extraordinary request for Dirk. He replies, 'You mean I don't do as much as you?' She doesn't understand what he's reacting to, but he grew up in a world defined by emotional distance and scarcity—where everything was measured. The kind of family where the price of every gift was compared. There's no concept of the bigger picture. That idea of 'together' is foreign to him. When you come from such different backgrounds, you each bring something extraordinary into the relationship. And that can shatter the illusion of the warm, safe home you've built together."

The *extraordinary* is what momentarily pulls us out of the safety of connection. The comfort of mutual understanding is disrupted. Difference introduces a sense of insecurity.

Everyone has habits and routines. In any relationship, differences in background, habits, or sensitivities naturally lead to tension. That's normal. It's part of being in a relationship. Two people bring two different worlds. Even simple things—like whether or not you have fixed seats at the table—can become sites of tension. Learning to live with someone different means adjusting, and that adjustment always carries some stress.

So, couples naturally introduce difference into each other's lives, and with that comes a level of tension they must learn to manage. But the pressure doesn't just come from within. It also comes from without—what we call *external stressors*. These, too, can disrupt the ordinary and add pressure to a relationship.

Lieven: "External stress can come from migration, financial problems, health issues, job loss, grief, family conflicts—even something like having children. Just imagine the tension when dealing with a runaway teenager in the house. These are the realities from outside that strike at the couple. So, every couple has to manage pressure from two sources: the extraordinary they bring to each other, and the stress imposed from outside. In both cases, this pressure introduces stress into the relationship, increasing the partners' need for support from each other. And yet, ironically, in the middle of that stress, people are often less capable of offering the attuned support the other needs. That creates a very human but significant tension. How partners deal with this sets the tone for how they cope together. And this pattern is universal."

Dealing with difference

When faced with the tension that the extraordinary brings to a couple, there are two common reactions: some people tend to step backward, while others tend to step forward. Those who step backward are more likely to respond with thoughts like, "I'll wait it out. I'll let it pass." Those who step forward react by saying, "We need to talk about this. We have to analyze it, think it through, and address it." This dynamic places partners in specific roles. In emotionally focused therapy (EFT), these are called the *withdrawn* position and the *pursuing* position—where one partner is more likely to seek distance when tension arises, and the other is more likely to seek closeness. There is nothing inherently wrong with either way of responding. However, when both partners become increasingly stuck in these opposing positions, difficulties often escalate. The resulting sense of powerlessness can become overwhelming. It can grow so intense that people may do anything to find peace or to reach the other person. This is the moment when violence can begin to emerge.

Jef: "I'll illustrate the development of this pattern with an example. When you go to sleep and undress, many people commonly leave their dirty laundry where it falls for a while or place it in a corner, then put it in the laundry basket the next morning. Others, however, find it perfectly normal to toss their dirty laundry directly into the basket immediately. Depending on your background and personality, there is a difference. As Lieven said, differences—and therefore tension—are inevitable within a couple. These tensions can range from very small things to the big issues of life. That makes sense. It is both bizarre and entirely normal that socks lying in the corner of a room can eventually lead to intense conflict. Or using each other's toothbrush. Or buying chocolate from a more expensive brand instead of the supermarket's house brand. Or whether to put a coat on the kids before they go outside to play. People argue fiercely over countless small matters. Of course, conflicts don't explode the first time a sock is left lying around or the first comment is made. It's about the accumulation. Even then, it's not really about laundry, toothbrushes, or shopping. It's about the loss of safety and security. 'If I leave my socks here and you get so angry… what does that say about who I am to you? Wasn't I that one special person for you? Then how is it that I suddenly become a deep disappointment in your eyes?' Or vice versa: 'If I ask you 20 times to put the sock in the laundry basket and you still just drop it wherever you stand, how important am I to you? Ignoring those socks so many times feels like you are ignoring me. How evident is my care for you, and can I count on your care?' Doubt begins to creep in."

Socks may seem trivial, but they can spark escalating conflicts. That's why it makes sense to play out an argument like this in slow motion. Suddenly, you hear the sock say, "Am I not good enough for you?" Or, "Are you going to be there for me?" And if that's the case… "Do we still belong together?" So *beneath the dirty laundry lie attachment questions*. These are not trivial. They trigger panic. This is where a pattern of interaction begins to develop.

From many little socks to the big themes in life

Attachment questions are not neatly packaged. We have to search for them beneath everyday conflicts. Of course, we don't mean a one-off occurrence, but rather frequent repetition or the accumulation of small differences. It is important to convey that these questions and the accompanying panic are equally present beneath the big, important issues. In those cases, repetition isn't even necessary.

Lieven: "For example, I think of a partner who suddenly becomes extremely angry with their young son and spanks him. That affects the other partner and provokes fierce reactions. Raising and caring for children is a topic that quickly evokes strong emotions. The same goes for health or money—these themes immediately carry a lot of intensity. 'I was so sick that I thought I was going to die, and you just kept working…' Those kinds of experiences. Or consider money: one partner spends freely, while the other grew up in poverty and learned to be very careful. 'If you throw our money away so quickly, I don't feel safe anymore. I fear losing our basic security. I'm afraid we'll lose everything we've built.' Or, 'If you give in so easily to our teenager, you'll jeopardize his future. He'll never learn perseverance, won't get a degree, and will lose many opportunities.' Friendships can evoke the same feelings: 'When I mispronounced a word, your friend laughed at me in front of everyone—and you laughed along. You know how ashamed I am of my dyslexia. You didn't stand up for me. I suddenly felt so alone. Even you abandoned me.' That is immediately very frightening. In that sense, it differs from minor differences."

Both the repeated small, seemingly trivial issues and the major life themes can create a buildup of conflict and lead to violence. In both cases, the question is whether the underlying attachment layer is activated. This determines the intensity of the reactions. 'Are you there for me? Am I good enough? Do I belong?' The more—and the more vehemently—these questions are answered negatively, the greater the emotional intensity and the more intense the conflicts become. Then escalation, and thus violence, is not far away.

Jef: "The couples who come to us often recount that small incident that suddenly becomes the straw that breaks the camel's back, and one partner says, 'Enough!' while the other wonders, 'What is this really about? Are we really fighting so fiercely over a sock?' What we aim to do as couples therapists is repeatedly separate the meaning of the argument from the sock itself. This helps partners express which attachment question has been triggered. Partners can easily see hundreds of socks lying around and be annoyed without becoming entangled in conflict. Or they can discuss and disagree over their children's future, caring for a sick parent, or other significant matters without losing each other in arguments. That also happens. In those cases, the underlying attachment issues are apparently not as strongly activated. Or partners manage to talk about them spontaneously with each other."

A predictable course unfolds

There are three ways the underlying attachment questions can be awakened: repeated small differences within the couple, differences or misunderstandings on the big themes of life, or major external stressors that put pressure on the relationship. Any of these can trigger that primary fear: "Am I important? Do I matter? Am I valuable? Am I good enough? Do I belong? Will we make it?" When that panic arises, partners need a great deal of reassurance from each other. When reassurance is lacking, the pain cuts deeply. No couple is exempt from this. Everyone encounters these questions and fears in one way or another. It is normal. Depending on which question awakens most strongly in you, there is a predictable pattern in your responses—and thus in the course the conflict takes, even when violence is involved. That same predictability applies there as well.

Jef: "If we make this concrete using our example of socks, it doesn't really matter where the story starts. There is no single person to blame or moment to pinpoint. But to outline a narrative, I'll begin with the partner who has been hearing repeated comments—let's say that's you. You've heard several times: 'That's not cool. That makes me nervous. Just throw that in the laundry basket already.' At the umpteenth angry glance, as you're about to take off your socks, you start to feel, 'Maybe you don't really like me that much after all.' Then one evening, when suddenly it bursts out, 'God-dammit! How many times do I have to ask? It's not that hard!' you're startled. Immediately afterward, you mutter, 'You can't be serious… how can you get that angry over a sock?' That anxious feeling of not being good enough usually first emerges as a kind of inner indignation. Some people express that indignation openly—that's when it no longer stays inside. Then a fire ignites quickly: 'Why do you always have to whine about such trivial things?' 'Why are such small things too much for you?' That kind of bickering begins. But many others keep mumbling and cursing inwardly."

Lieven: "What often accompanies this is fear: 'I don't understand. What does he mean? What have I done wrong again?' Doubt, fear, confusion. 'I want so badly to do the right thing, but I don't know what that is. It can't be about that sock. It can't be. But what then?' This feeling of being trapped is immediate. Or as Crosby, Stills, Nash & Young sing, 'It increases my paranoia. Like looking in the mirror and seeing a police car.' I know that feeling well—the tension when a police car stops you, and you don't know what you've done wrong. This tension is not unfamiliar to people in the withdrawing position."

So, it all begins with a comment—spoken or nonverbal, like a raised eyebrow or a piercing glance. A comment about the little things or the very big things, and what the other person means to us. From there, the pattern literally and figuratively becomes visible in the interactions.

When one of those three pressures weighs on a couple, it is inevitable that one partner will eventually gather courage and start speaking up. There's a big difference—a significant, intense event has happened, and we need to address it. Then one of you begins talking about socks, children, or financial difficulties.

Jef: "When people start talking about these things, it's usually not gentle or mild—there's tension. Then the other partner typically reacts in one of two ways: they either respond with protest, or they fall silent and withdraw. When both partners start talking and protesting more clearly at each other, you get a symmetrical escalation.

More common, though, is that one partner steps forward and the other steps back. Then one partner tries to discuss socks, children, or a sick parent, while the other hears only, 'I'm not doing it right.' It's quite logical, then, that this partner doesn't know how to respond, so they avoid the topic, remain silent, or change the subject. On the surface, it looks like silence or 'problem-solving.' But rarely is there a real conversation about what's actually going on between them. The question, '*What is going on between us?*' remains unspoken, hanging in the air. That causes frustration in the partner trying to talk. Although that partner often does not clearly express the feelings beneath the socks—for example, '*I feel like I'm not important to you*'—they mainly focus on the practical side."

... or you hear each other

Before we explore this conflict pattern more deeply, let's consider another possible course of interaction. When one partner raises an issue, the other may actually hear them. Someone brings something up, the other picks up on it, and together they genuinely discuss what is happening. In this scenario, partners hear and understand each other. They don't have to agree, but they feel they're not alone and can talk about it together. This is very powerful. Such moments happen in every couple. In a way, this might be the most wonderful path. There are many reasons why it is difficult to understand each other. It's not obvious that a sock represents feelings of importance, being good enough, and belonging. Being able to speak in a way that touches on that deeper layer—that's special. And it does happen. When it does, a feeling of 'Finally!' grows, and together you build your home as a couple. That is very powerful.

The other moments stand alongside these—times when difficult issues arise but you don't spontaneously arrive at an understanding conversation.

Lieven: "So it's not all conflict and tension. Couples sometimes get tangled up only after 10 years, or they have periods when things don't work out, then suddenly another period when they reconnect. That's exactly why it's so difficult when, at another time or about a different topic, you suddenly find that you can't manage to talk about it. That hurts and induces feelings of vulnerability. Then you start sounding angrier and sharper, which makes it even more painful. Somewhere inside, you think, 'Wow, we handle things well. We're a good team.' Until suddenly you reach a place where it doesn't work anymore, where you lose that sense somewhat. That's frightening and painful."

The pattern takes shape

Returning to the partner who wants to discuss something: they do not do this for pleasure but out of concern for the relationship. Something has been lingering in the air for a while, and both partners have let it be until one of them decides, "We have to address this." There are many small or moderately significant issues involved. External pressures weigh on the relationship. Sometimes one partner initiates the conversation; other times, the other does. Early in a relationship, there usually isn't a clear pattern to this. But after some time—or in certain cases—the act of discussing becomes stuck. This occurs when underlying attachment needs or fears are triggered but go unnoticed by the other partner. When this happens repeatedly, a pattern emerges in their interactions. This pattern has both an outer and an inner dimension.

Jef: "Exactly how this happens varies greatly from couple to couple, but I will try to outline what often occurs. If one partner eventually finds the courage or the relational care to bring up the issue, it is both difficult and exciting to do so—and equally tense to hear such a thing as the other partner. Inside, one might think, 'Oh, dear!' If you struggle with the question, 'Am I good enough?' you are likely to interpret your partner's attempt at conversation as criticism: 'See, I have failed in your eyes.' What often prevents people from discussing what's on the table is that they do not hear the message being conveyed but instead hear, 'My partner thinks I'm not good enough—again.' This perception inevitably activates your attachment strategy: withdrawing, avoiding conversation, and shielding yourself. These strategies can be very effective. Internally, you might feel frustrated, but you think, 'If I express this, things will only get worse, so I'd rather avoid the conversation.'

At that moment, the partner who brought up the issue notices, 'I tried to discuss something, and now you've shut down—I can't feel you anymore!' This doesn't make the original problem any bigger, but it does make *our* shared problem enormous. 'I wanted to solve this together, and I can't.' The question on this partner's mind is often, '*Are you there for me?*' The avoidance that follows the attempt to talk answers that question negatively: 'You're not here. This is too difficult, apparently. I'm not important to you.' That question intensifies in the silence: 'Can we continue together? Do we still belong together if I don't matter to you?' The longer that question goes unanswered, the more emotions swell, making the need to discuss it even stronger. "That's when one partner might say, 'You know, that's always how it is! It's not just the socks. With the dishes, you do the same—you never put your plate in the dishwasher; it always stays on the kitchen counter. Or with the kids—if they say something about their homework, you just shut down.' You reinforce your message by listing examples of when you felt your partner wasn't there for you.

Because you start listing these examples so quickly and vehemently, using absolute terms like 'never' and 'always,' the couple is likely to become even more stuck. Those words—'never,' 'always'—and all the examples make the pain on the other side grow as well: 'Wait, if it's already about the socks, you think I don't love you anymore. I want to protest, but when I do, I hear that not only at night, when I take off my clothes, are you disappointed in me, but that every breakfast, lunch, and dinner you think the same when I put my plate on the counter. That I don't immediately help with the children also bothers you. And these things don't just bother you today—you apparently always find them troublesome?!'

So the question, 'Am I good enough for you?' is answered loudly in the negative. The emotions involved are intensely painful and provoke so much protest that the best way to cope seems to be to avoid feeling them. 'I'll just go to work, and when I come back, it will be over.' Or, 'I'll take the dog for a walk around the block, and it will cool down.' Don't feel too much. Of course, this is not helpful to the other partner. This is where the negative response to the underlying attachment question grows."

Lieven: "If you get stuck in this cycle regularly, an even greater fear arises for both partners: 'We can't communicate with each other. *What does that say about our relationship?*' When that fear emerges, we no longer dare to discuss issues openly. Instead, concerns appear camouflaged or behind the firm armor we place on the relationship table. We no longer dare to bring up concerns gently and clearly, thinking, 'We can't do that anyway.' The body begins to speak loudly—the tone of voice, facial expressions, tightened mouths.

The partner trying to initiate or continue the discussion may not always perceive the depth of these signals—or they do but try to suppress their feelings for fear that things will go wrong again. So, the conversation quickly becomes fraught with tension. Then the feeling arises, 'We used to communicate so well, and now? We can't even talk about socks anymore.' The panic intensifies, as does the urge to keep (disguising) the conversation.

Inside the partner pursuing the connection is a sense of loneliness. 'I feel alone. I need you but can't find you. I'm afraid you won't respond. I need support but don't yet know how to ask for it.' Because of the fear that the other won't be there, their words become harsher. This is the reverse logic of emotions: the more support I need, the more afraid and insecure I am to show it. The more afraid I am, the angrier and 'stronger' my words become. Often, we humans have not learned how to say what we need. *The more dangerous and compelling the need, the more camouflaged the expression.* If you ask for what you need, you risk rejection. So it's easier to say, 'You never hug me!' than, 'Will you hug me sometime? I need it.' To the latter, your partner can say no, which leaves you more vulnerable than if you communicate a judgment about your partner. In the discussing position, we often don't realize that what we say sounds like an attack—that we are pointing at the other person.

The partner more likely to withdraw often thinks, 'Why do we have to argue so much? I don't know what else to do or say.' Frequently, this stems from never having learned how to argue safely at home. So fear grows on this side as well."

From fear to panic

The pattern that develops between couples through many repeated interactions begins to take shape. To understand how these awkward yet familiar exchanges can escalate into a spiral of violence, we need to consider the missing piece of the puzzle: intensity. The fear that arises from the awakened attachment questions grows into panic as the emotional distance increases. The stronger the underlying emotions, the more intense the reactions become. Both partners dig in deeper behind their protective barriers, which causes them to hear and understand each other less and less. Below, we outline what this looks like in concrete terms.

Jef: “This entire dynamic applies to many small examples, but imagine what it looks like for the major issues in a relationship. Then the urgency to speak up grows, as does the danger involved in speaking. ‘*We really need to talk about this*! Our relationship is at risk.’ For people in the pursuing, discussing position, these moments are filled with strong emotions and rapid speech. They sound the alarm—and understandably so. When you feel cracks forming in the foundation of your house because there’s so much distance, and you can’t fix it by talking, you don’t remain calm. Instead, you think, ‘This is a big problem, and it must be addressed quickly and forcefully!’ The discussion that follows is not necessarily the problem—perhaps it is even necessary. However, the intensity of the discussion often backfires. The forcefulness and rapid pace of the conversation are rarely well-received by the other partner. Then it doesn’t feel like the relationship has a problem; it feels like *I* am the problem. This is where misunderstandings between couples arise. What is heard with great intensity is, ‘You’ve failed! She’s disappointed in me. I’m not good enough!’ This creates a lot of painful feelings inside, which then invite one to retreat behind a shield or bunker.

At the same time, if your partner is saying with great intensity, ‘We MUST discuss this TOGETHER!’ but all you hear through the vehemence is, ‘I’m clearly the reason everything is going wrong here,’ you crawl further into your bunker. Your partner then feels, ‘You don’t want to talk to me. I’m not that important. My needs and burdens don’t matter to you.’

A typical example goes like this:

> ‘What’s going on?’
> ‘Nothing.’
> ‘But you’ve been so quiet for days.’
> ‘No, really, nothing’s wrong.’

Behind that ‘nothing,’ someone hidden in their bunker is feeling, ‘My partner is missing something in this relationship. Why is it never good enough? I’m trying so hard already. But clearly something is wrong. It’s better not to show myself because if I do, I’ll feel even more that I can’t give her what she needs.’ The other partner, sitting with frustration, thinks, ‘Tell me what it is, so we can deal with it together. If you can’t tell me, who am I to you?’

When your partner seems to drift further away as you try to reach them, you will eventually try anything to break through and feel like a partner who matters. You make a firm fist and bang on the door of their bunker. If there's no response for a long time, you start saying anything to be heard or felt: 'There really is a problem in this relationship! When will you see that? If you don't take responsibility, things will fall apart. Come out of your hole now!' At that point, the other person doesn't hear, '*Come out of your bunker, I need you.*' Instead, they hear, 'That bunker is the problem, but it's part of me—that's who I am. So, I'm the problem.' Then there are only two options: bunker deeper or push the other away by placing a strong cannon on your bunker."

Lieven: "That cannon often starts with: 'If you say it like that, I'm not listening.' This is one of the most familiar defensive phrases to all that vehement pursuing. In response, the partner who wanted to discuss something naturally feels, 'I'm the one trying to start the conversation, and apparently that's not right. Now my tone is wrong too. Suddenly, it's all about me. But when will we talk about what really matters? When will I be allowed to say something about those socks?!'

Another common defensive phrase is, 'If you ask one more time what's going on, then something will go on!' This reminds us that the partner who withdraws does not always do so silently. Sometimes the withdrawal looks quite fierce on the outside."

The tipping toward violence

What we describe here is a dynamic familiar to all couples. Fortunately, many couples are eventually able to reconnect. These are the couples who, at some point, realize they can let go of surface-level issues—like arguments about socks—and begin to safely express the emotions underneath. When they're able to talk about these deeper feelings, conflicts can be resolved.

But sometimes the conflicts persist. They may last so long, or the underlying issues may be so significant and painful, or external pressures on the couple may be so intense, that they cannot find a way out. In such cases, couples can become stuck in a pattern that lasts for months or even years. When this happens frequently or intensely, it creates a fertile ground where the shift toward partner violence can become a dangerously small step.

Jef: "To understand more deeply how this pattern can escalate into partner violence, let's start by 'talking about it.' Imagine this cycle has been repeating for months. One partner—typically the person in the pursuing position—is trying to bring problems into the open and has already tried again and again to make it clear that something needs to change in the relationship. But all they've encountered is the other partner saying, 'I'm fine,' while retreating further into emotional isolation. Powerlessness builds: 'If you don't see the problem, then I'm alone with it.' It begins to feel as if the foundation of your home is cracking, and panic sets in. Over time, your words become stronger and more direct because nothing else seems to get through. You begin using absolutes like 'never' and 'always.' But the firmer and clearer your words become, the more distant your partner seems, and the more isolated you feel.

Eventually, the powerlessness becomes so overwhelming that you resort to more extreme expressions. The metaphorical fist knocking on the door of your partner's emotional bunker is no longer just a strong word—it becomes physical. At some point, your partner feels so distant that it's as if you've been completely abandoned, as though you *no longer matter to them at all*. In desperation, you do whatever you can to reestablish contact, to make clear that something deeply important is at stake. Suddenly, you grab the vase from the table and throw it at their head."

Lieven: "Those are often the moments when the partner in the 'bunker' says, 'I'm out. Even my bunker isn't safe anymore, so I'm leaving.' This may look like a total emotional shutdown—hours or days of silence, refusing to respond. It can also mean literally leaving the room or the house: getting in the car and driving away. Unsurprisingly, this is often the point when the last thread of self-control snaps for the pursuing partner. The conscious desire to connect with the other person turns into something raw and primal—a desperate internal voice shouting, 'Don't leave me! This is the end. If you walk out now, you'll never come back! I'll be alone forever.' It's pure panic and helplessness screaming, 'You can't leave. You mustn't leave.' This is the moment when powerlessness turns into the use of power: you begin using force to keep the other person from leaving. You block the door. You pull them out of the car. You scratch them—not to hurt them, but to make them feel that you're still there, to show them it's hurting you too much to let them go."

Fighting for your existence

Violence has taken hold, fueled by panic and helplessness. The emotional state in that moment closely resembles the separation anxiety seen in small children when they're left with someone unfamiliar for the first time. Perhaps you know the phase: you drop your child off at daycare, and he roars and cries at the door as you walk away. It's a profound experience of losing the reassuring presence of the caregiver—the loss of the long-awaited *finally*, of the safe home.

At this point, it's no longer about socks or dishes left on the counter. It's not even about the bigger themes—like parenting disagreements, the pain of a miscarriage, the heavy burden of job loss, or caring for a parent with psychiatric issues. What it's really about is: *I'm losing you.*

That feeling can be deeply destabilizing and overwhelming. In response, a person may do whatever it takes to maintain some form of connection. We see this in children's behavior: "Better negative attention than no attention at all." Like the three-year-old who starts biting when he feels unseen or unheard—he acts out to provoke a response. Similarly, one might think: *My partner is so angry and withdrawn… they're never coming back. I can't let them leave. I have to stop them.* The panic runs even deeper: *If you don't respond, I cease to exist. If you leave, I will fall to pieces. I won't be truly alive anymore.* People often describe this as a near-death feeling. *I need an anchor, or we both sink—and I sink.* It's profoundly existential. That's the depth behind the intensity of the reaction.

Jef: "In that moment, you are overwhelmed. There's deep frustration, profound powerlessness, and an intense fear of abandonment—the terrifying sense of losing your worth, your very being. In such a cocktail of emotions, it's not surprising that people sometimes act out in extreme ways, even violently. *It becomes a fight for connection*—a fight for love. Hitting, scratching, cursing, kicking… doing whatever it takes to wake the other up, to pull them out of the bunker and reestablish some kind of contact. 'Are you still there? Are you still with me? Are you still there *for* me?' Taking the car keys, smashing a phone, locking the door—these are all violent acts, but underneath, they are desperate attempts to prevent abandonment. Even if it's harmful, it comes from a place of *I need to feel that there is still a connection—that I still exist in relationship with you.*"

No matter how far violence may seem from your character or values, it's astonishing how many people can reach a point where something takes over, and they cross a line. When that emotional chain reaction takes hold, people do things that seem to contradict the love they feel—yet paradoxically, it reveals how essential their partner's love truly is. The human need for connection both sustains love and, at times, endangers it.

Lieven: "At the same time, of course, there's someone on the other side—someone entrenched in the bunker who is also suffering. He or she feels the words of that angry, demanding voice—reaching out, trying to make contact—pounding down like an unrelenting storm. The partner isn't giving up, and that storm feels overwhelming. The experience is something like: *'Whoa! What's coming at me? I'm drowning in these emotions. I can't take this anymore.'* So you continually say, 'Stop! Just Stop!'—at first silently, then more audibly and clearly. You try anything to make it stop because it feels dangerous, both to yourself and to the relationship.

When you keep asking for it to stop and it doesn't, you begin to withdraw—to escape. That withdrawal, of course, is exactly the moment that frightens your partner even more, causing them to try even harder to keep you close. People in this withdrawn position often describe a mental shutdown: 'I have to get out of here, or I'll lose control!' And if someone is halted in the midst of such a fierce and overwhelming emotional state, it's not uncommon for them to resort to violence.

At that moment, the only thought in the mind of the withdrawn person is: 'This has to stop.' There is something about it that feels life-threatening. *'If it doesn't stop, I'll suffocate.'* Many people describe it as a sensation of running out of air, about to explode, vision going black, a fuse blowing. They shift into survival mode, seeking calm—because somewhere inside, they believe: 'If this continues, I will explode. If I stay in this conversation, I'll become extremely angry. And then things will really spiral out of control. That would be much worse.' So they retreat, close off, and bunker down. Outwardly, that may appear calm or even icy, but internally, it's exhausting. Containing that tension, holding back that immense emotional energy—it works for a while. But eventually, that pressure also erupts, often unpredictably. Then there may be an outburst—a shove, a strike—from this side."

The existential dimension is evident in both positions. The aggression is so painful, so devoid of love—and yet, for both partners, it is deeply rooted in the desperate cry: "I need the other in order to exist!" For one partner, that need is for the other to be at rest with them; for the other, it's for the partner to stay in contact with them. But from both we hear: 'If the other disappears in this way, I cease to exist.' When you peel back the dynamics, what you find in both positions is a longing for Being. "'I need you to Be there,' and when that Being is threatened, a powerful—and unfortunately destructive—force is activated."

Two types of aggression

There are two positions in which individuals are at high risk of turning to violence: the pursuing position and the withdrawing position. In both, the emotional intensity becomes so overwhelming that it spills over into violent behavior. While the aggression can be equally intense in both cases, it reflects different meanings and expresses different needs. We therefore distinguish between two types of aggression: distance-seeking and proximity-seeking aggression.

Jef: "The person in the withdrawing position does everything they can to stop the tension. The violence this person resorts could be described as 'stop violence.' We refer to it as space-seeking or *distance-seeking aggression*. The aim is to halt the flood of words, which internally sound like: 'Not good enough, failed, you're a disappointment!' This leads to a profound loss of self and security, creating an urgent need to end the situation. At the same time, you don't want to become angry, don't want to cause harm, and you want to protect the foundation of your relationship. So, you put in a tremendous effort to manage both the overwhelming internal tension and the stream of external blame. The internal logic becomes: 'I have to do something to stop this, but I can't do anything—because if I let go of this feeling, everything will fall apart.' It's an excruciating tension. Paradoxically, this distance-seeking strategy, along with the partner's reaction to it, pushes you so far into helplessness that the only perceived escape is a violent outburst—pushing your partner away, silencing them, even physically restraining them. Anything to make it stop. It's incredibly complex."

Lieven: "The other partner, driven to talk, connect, and restore closeness, may then shift into what we call *proximity-seeking aggression*.

As you can imagine, when these two collide, it becomes deeply destructive. The couple harms one another emotionally and, at times, physically—even though underneath, the motivation is love. These are two people hurting each other because they love each other intensely and are suffering profoundly from the loss of the other's loving eyes."

A house on the verge of collapse

When your very sense of self is at stake—precisely because the relationship matters so deeply—it is possible for anyone to end up in violent escalations. Discussions of partner violence often focus on power, but in the vast majority of cases, the core issue is powerlessness. It is the desperation of feeling, "I can't get this across, and yet our foundation is cracking," or "That feeling of finally being close is slipping away—I'm losing you." This leads to panic, speechlessness, and an overwhelming emotional state that feels inescapable. Letting go feels like losing yourself.

Jef: "It sounds outrageously loud and looks terribly ugly, but it says only one thing: I am fighting for love—to find the other again, to find myself, and to find our 'us.' Without that, I can't exist. But this fight is expressed through such a torrent of words and actions that it generates intense insecurity in the other person. They experience it as: 'She doesn't understand that I'm trying so hard to do right by her. Everything I do seems to make it worse. What else can I do? There's no way out!' Or: 'The peaceful, safe home we built together is cracking.' Then you try to remain as still as possible in that home because any movement might cause it to collapse. But that's almost impossible when the other person is shouting, pushing, or throwing things. Your panic rises: 'It's all going to fall apart!' And your mind screams: 'This has to stop—at all costs!' The more you try to stay still, hide in a corner, or move away, the louder your partner shouts, 'Can't you see this part needs support?!' You think, 'I can't respond—if I prop it up, the whole thing might collapse. Stop shaking this house, woman! This is going terribly wrong!' Here, you have two people caught in completely different perceptions of the same thing: *the loss of self and/or the relationship*. And when the repeated cry of 'Stop!' isn't heard, tragically, it often leads to the use of force to silence the other. 'If I can make my partner stop talking, our house will be safe again.' These moments are often explosive and deeply painful. This is how people become completely stuck and lose each other."

The chicken or the egg

So far, we have outlined the course of escalating conflict as if distance-seeking aggression always follows pursuing or proximity-seeking aggression. Of course, this is not always the case. Violence can emerge on both sides, on one side only, or on neither side. But when it does appear, we consistently recognize these movements, interactions, and buildup beneath it.

Lieven: "Anything is possible. Distance-seeking aggression always follows pursuing sounds, movements, or expressions. Likewise, proximity-seeking aggression always follows withdrawing movements or expressions. It's really a circular process. You cannot pinpoint a clear beginning. By the way, it does not always escalate into aggression on both sides. Similarly, one partner may exhibit proximity-seeking aggression without the other partner resorting to violence. One partner can simply display distance-seeking behavior, remain silent, or continue to withdraw without using violence. Alternatively, one partner may continue to pursue but shut down in response to the other partner's distance-seeking violence, or continue pursuing without using violence."

Jef: "Moreover, these patterns and positions have nothing to do with gender. We know this from the PASK study of John Hamel (Hamel & Nicholls, 2007). The Partner Abuse State of Knowledge Project is an ongoing comprehensive, peer-reviewed research synthesis on intimate partner violence led by John Hamel and colleagues, summarizing findings across prevalence, risk factors, intervention outcomes, and policy (Domestic Violence Research, 2016). This research tells us that both women and men can engage in violence. Both can assume either of the two positions and thus exhibit proximity-seeking or distance-seeking aggression. For example, we observe the same patterns and prevalence of violence in LGBTQI+ relationships. In heterosexual couples experiencing partner violence, both partners use violence in 6 out of 10 cases. The same statistic applies to male–male and female–female relationships, where we observe the same *bi-directionality*, as we call it. So, it is less about gender and more about the extent to which attachment issues are activated. To what degree is the question 'Are you there for me?' or 'Am I good enough?' increasingly answered with 'No!' during interactions? It is at that point that extreme behaviors emerge—used either to connect or to regain peace of mind for oneself and the relationship."

Lieven: "For completeness, I would like to add that there is one domain where gender makes an important difference: *physical force*. Generally, when men resort to physical violence, it has a greater impact because men are often physically stronger, resulting in more severe injuries. This violence tends to be less casual, affecting the sense of (in)safety. However, the physical and psychological impact of violence by women against men also has significant negative effects that cannot be ignored. Another factor to consider is socioeconomic status. Many cultures, societies, and situations still render women more socioeconomically vulnerable, and that inequality also affects (in)security. At the same time, in cases of bi-directional violence, we often observe that women can be much more powerful and more likely to engage in physical violence than popular portrayals suggest."

So, the stereotypical image of partner violence featuring a narcissistic male perpetrator exerting power over a helpless female victim does not represent the daily reality of this issue. The reality for most couples is much more nuanced. As we noted earlier, only a small percentage of cases involve intimate terrorism—where power is central. Furthermore, almost anything is possible in terms of the direction and form of violence. What is crucial is that this is an interaction in which both parties suffer, each fighting for connection in their own way.

Symmetrical escalation

The interaction patterns described in this chapter involve a back-and-forth dynamic between someone in the pursuing position and someone in the withdrawn position. Of course, there are couples in which both partners employ the same attachment strategy. What do the dynamics look like when both partners are in the pursuing position or both are in the withdrawn position?

Jef: "Those couples certainly exist. However, when it comes to partner violence, both partners will only be in the pursuing position temporarily. At some point during an escalation, one person almost always feels, 'Wow, this is dangerous!' That person becomes afraid of themselves or the other and shifts toward more withdrawn behavior, seeking a 'Stop!'"

Lieven: "Research highlights another important aspect of violence in relationships. Let me explain. People involved in mutual violence often say to each other, 'You don't understand me. You're not there for me.' They blame one another, and arguments escalate suddenly into pushing or hitting. When this happens, many couples feel, 'We crossed a line. We don't want this anymore.' In such cases, violence can serve a functional purpose. It signals a boundary that helps stop the escalation. During the cooling-down phase, the couple comes together and acknowledges, 'That was too violent, right? We don't want that. What made it so violent? It wasn't about those socks, was it? Maybe it was about feeling like we weren't taking good care of each other. For me, it was about not feeling good enough in your eyes. What about you?' These are couples who literally or figuratively punched a hole in the wall during a fierce argument but then repaired it together. In these cases, violence is not destructive; it activates something that binds and regulates the relationship.

However, when incidents of violence become very intense, one partner often decides, 'I'm not going to fight anymore. It's too dangerous. I was afraid it would go completely wrong. I feared I might do something to you that I truly don't want to.' Or, 'This was so scary. You frightened me. I suddenly feared you might really destroy me. I don't dare to show myself fully anymore, and I'm not going to let you get that close. It's too dangerous.' Or, 'I heard you say such vehement things about me during the argument that I suddenly feel very deeply that you no longer think I'm good enough.' These reactions represent two ways a person *shifts into the withdrawn position*, either to protect themselves or to protect the relationship.

Paradoxically, this makes things even more intense or frightening, because it becomes even harder to come together safely. One person takes a step forward while the other steps back, starting a difficult-to-break cycle. So, to answer the question: symmetrical or equal escalations are simply not sustainable."

We rarely observe two partners both in the withdrawn position when discussing partner violence. This does not mean it doesn't exist. We don't often see these couples in therapy, but experience shows that couples stuck in the withdrawn position can also escalate into violence. Two mechanisms explain this.

The most obvious occurs when a couple has been stuck in the familiar dynamic of pursuer and withdrawer for some time, but at one point experiences excessive danger of violence. As a result, the pursuing partner *retreats into withdrawal out of fear*. (This parallels the movement seen when two partners are both pursuing and one shifts to withdrawal due to fear.) All feelings of lack, loss, hurt, and associated frustration are bunker-like-protected to preserve the relationship. People can maintain this for surprisingly long periods until the proverbial straw breaks the camel's back and violent escalation occurs.

The second mechanism involves two people who meet in the withdrawn position—like two turtles cautiously maintaining distance. These partners typically have very limited language for expressing their inner world, desires, needs, or differences between them. In growing into adulthood, withdrawal was their only safe place. It was safe but often lonely. This dynamic creates a paradox: they yearn for contact as adults but simultaneously fear it.

In the first dynamic, withdrawal–withdrawal represents a closing phase in the relational pattern. In the second, it is a starting point based on what was familiar in childhood.

Jef: "Imagine this as a large dam people have built to hold in all their feelings—a dam that silences those feelings into a vast reservoir. External factors, such as difficult life events or substance abuse, can cause a sudden breach. Then, a huge volume of water is released with tremendous force, sweeping away everything in its path. This is where violence takes place. The released energy can mean a desire to reach and cling to the other person as well as a desire to push that person away. Extending the dam metaphor, the contained need for closeness breaks loose, or the force of the released water is used to maintain a familiar distance. In these couples, there is always a complex combination of both needs: the water pushes them toward one another and simultaneously pushes the other away."

Typically, couples stuck in this dynamic try to repair the crack or break in the dam as quickly as possible to prevent further damage. They are frightened by the violence and, although they long for closeness somewhere inside, it still feels safer to maintain familiar distance. They would rather endure the immense pressure of a full reservoir than risk being flooded by the force of released water. No one taught them how to navigate the chaos of their inner world or how to manage the floodwaters safely. So, they keep returning to the silence of their familiar reservoirs.

Conclusion: intense love

We began this chapter with a slide we created many years ago: partner violence = common conflicts × 10. Since then, the meaning of this statement has become much clearer. The progression of conflicts, whether repeated trivial issues, painful major themes, or strong external pressures, generates tension because these conflicts also trigger underlying attachment concerns. This dynamic is universal to all couples, with or without violence. Our responses to these tense attachment questions, either stepping forward (pursuing, wanting to discuss) or stepping back (withdrawing, remaining silent, and waiting for it to pass), are true for all couples.

It takes little imagination to see how these two steps set in motion a dance that can become very intense. The difference lies in the degree of intensity. Some couples overcome the intensity on their own, sometimes even working through it to achieve a deeper understanding of each other. At the same time, many couples do not overcome it, and the anxious tension grows into a panic so existential that they feel compelled to fight for their very existence within the relationship.

The idea that violence can be so closely intertwined with love is frightening. Perhaps this is why, as a society, we prefer to place it in a separate box. We don't want violence to enter our homes, families, or relationships, so we push it toward abnormality and deviance. Yet the buildup—the way an argument develops and unfolds—is so universal. The move toward violence suddenly seems understandable and even logical when we feel a powerful need for a safe other.

Those who suddenly find themselves in a place where love has been overtaken by violence often ask themselves, "What is wrong with me that we ended up here?" At other times, the question sounds like, "What is wrong with my partner that we ended up here?" We humans tend to seek simple answers to complicated situations. That this is not a straightforward story is something we have clearly outlined in this conversation. In the next chapter, we will take a closer look at those last two questions.

Reflect and relate

Take a moment to pause and connect these ideas to your own experience.

The questions below are not meant to judge or define your relationship. They are an invitation to look at your own moves in conflict—what you do, what you feel, and what you long for underneath.

1. When you imagine looking at one of your typical (not yet escalated) arguments from a helicopter view, do you recognize yourself more in the *pursuing* or in the *withdrawing* position?

2. What fear lives beneath this outer behavior? Do you recognize the question "Am I good enough?" or rather "Are you there for me?"

3. Complete the following sentence in your own words and delete what doesn't apply:

4. "The more I feel that I'm not doing it right / that I'm on my own, the more I tend to ...... (withdrawing behavior) / ...... (pursuing behavior). The more I do that, the more my partner feels that I'm not there for them / they are not doing it right, and then they tend to ...... (pursuing behavior) / ...... (withdrawing behavior)."

5. When this loop keeps repeating, do you notice that your anger shows up to help you *reach* your partner (closeness-seeking aggression) or to *stop* the conflict (distance-seeking aggression)?

6. If you imagine talking to your partner about this, how would you describe this movement of seeking distance or seeking closeness in your own words?

References

Domestic Violence Research. (2016). *Partner abuse state of knowledge project.* https://domesticviolenceresearch.org/

Hamel, J., & Nicholls, T. L. (2007). *Family interventions in domestic violence: A handbook of gender-inclusive theory and treatment.* Springer.

4

IS SOMETHING WRONG WITH ME, YOU, OR US?

"When I look at the people and couples around me, I don't think anyone fights as violently as we do. Sometimes I mention it to friends, and I hear that everyone has their difficulties. It may look more peaceful on the outside than behind closed doors, but nowhere does it seem as bad as with us. That must mean something is wrong with us as a couple, right?"

"The way she can switch from being such an involved, warm, funny wife and mom to an angry, aggressive, abusive person who destroys so much… I'm shocked every time. There's no way to understand it. I've never experienced anything like that in a relationship. I think there's something really wrong with her."

"It's not normal that I feel so utterly rejected every time. She tells me repeatedly afterward that it's not personal, yet it feels that way each time—as if I'm a complete failure. What's worse: suddenly, I notice that I'm pinching her throat shut, and then I see fear in her eyes as she gasps for air. What kind of person am I to hurt the woman I love most like this? I am really messed up. I don't dare say this to anyone… They would all think I'm insane."

DOI: 10.4324/9781003683582-5

A quarter of all people experience partner violence at some point in their lives. Many more become caught up in escalating conflicts and are familiar with thoughts like these. Regularly ending up in heated arguments or experiencing partner violence leaves a mark. It affects how we see ourselves, our partner, and our relationship. It makes it harder to view the relationship with confidence. Doubts begin to creep in. The ground beneath you and your partner becomes unstable. This uncertainty is expressed in questions such as, "What's wrong with me? Is something wrong with my partner? Surely something must be wrong with our relationship?" In this chapter, we take a closer look at these questions.

Keep it simple

Most problems in life are complicated and that causes us some anxiety. Think of global warming or the traffic jams around Brussels or any other capital. When you try to find a solution to such problems, you get tangled up and tense, because if you move one piece of the puzzle, other pieces move too—and things can go wrong. Our brains panic in the face of complexity. To handle this, our brains use a clever trick: the more scared we feel, the simpler we want things to be. The more complicated the problem, the stronger our brain's urge to find a simple solution. Our brains naturally work by cause and effect. These two facts together make us humans look for a simple answer to complex problems—ideally one cause and one culprit. For example, when a train derailed in Greece recently, the first question on the news was, "Whose fault was that?" As if there could only be one cause.

We have this same tendency with psychological suffering and human misery. We tend to ask, "Who is sick?" and then look for diagnoses. It's no different with couples suffering from violence. Here too, the story is complex and creates a lot of tension and anxiety: I love you so much, yet we fight each other—that's confusing. So, there is a natural tendency to look for a simple answer with one guilty party. The pointing finger is born: "Is something wrong with me? Is something wrong with my partner? Is something wrong with us?"

Lieven: "In this book, we provide answers to several questions about partner violence and how it happens. We offer clear answers, but not simple ones. That goes against our brain's tendency when faced with a heavy topic like partner violence. The brain wants a simple yes or no, he / she / them or I. I remember something from Watzlawick in the 1980s. He was an Austrian-American psychologist, philologist, and world-renowned communication scholar, best known for his communication axioms. He learned us that when two things happen together, our brain wants to draw a straight line from A to B. That's how it works upstairs. We like to know who is to blame because it *gives the illusion that we know what to do next*. 'If we know the fault, we just fix it and the problem disappears.'

We see this same process in the people around the couple. They suffer because they see someone they love hurting. They feel powerless, ask many questions, and often feel fear… so they look for a simple cause and a culprit. That makes it easier to handle. For those around the couple, having a guilty party also protects them. If I know there is something wrong with you, then there is nothing wrong with me. That gives peace of mind. And when faced with something as overwhelming as violence between loved ones, *peace* of mind is very welcome.

But it's not that simple. For one, this affects a quarter of the population. You are not alone with this, so you are not weird or wrong because there is violence in your relationship. It is something you suffer from, so you want to understand it to do something about it. That is what we aim to do here. We want to give clear, but not simple answers in this book."

Jef: "Couples dealing with partner violence want clarity. They tend to want simple answers. We don't go along with that. We follow the logic of attachment theory here. Sometimes it seems simple, but it's not. The more you know, the more complex it becomes, and we cannot keep it simple. Attachment offers a framework that can bring clarity. So when the question arises, 'What's wrong with me or you or us?' we answer in a way that helps us understand what is happening between and within us, without looking for someone to blame. We take away the idea of 'fault'—without denying that bad things are happening and people are getting hurt. Of course, there are difficulties in the relationship and environment—that's the complexity. But it can't be traced to a single cause. Labels like 'narcissistic man' or 'borderline woman' do not bring clarity."

When people are caught in escalating conflicts, it is usually a threatening experience. Naturally, they—and their brains—need to understand what is happening to reduce the threat. Because our brain is organized to simplify cause and effect, this desire for peace and understanding often comes out in questions like, "Is something wrong with me, with you, or with us?" The wisdom behind these questions is that when you're stuck in painful, complex interactions, you seek solid ground. With this book, we want to offer that solid ground—a clear support that is not accusatory.

"Guess who?" as part of the conflict

The "one cause—one culprit" way of thinking makes perfect sense in the complex and confusing situation of partner violence. However, it would be dangerous to give a linear causal answer to such a question because there is something else peculiar about these kinds of questions: they arise from an interaction cycle—and they fuel it. These questions perpetuate the negative coupling dynamic.

Jef: "When your partner firmly tells you there is something wrong with you, you usually don't feel invited to show yourself openly to them. If you come to believe that there really is something wrong with your partner, it would be logical to want to make that clear so they can address it: 'It's because you spend so much time away with your friends that things go wrong between us,' or, 'It's because you expect too much that we're always fighting.' A response to this simple question will follow—one that only produces more of the same. If we decide something is wrong with us, then we are stuck with a big problem. That fear arises: can we continue together? That fear makes us anything but calm, of course, and it only fuels the tension in our conflicts. So, the questions, 'Is something wrong with you, with me, or with us?' are part of the interaction cycle."

Lieven: "In themselves, these are very logical questions that arise from our brain's need to simplify very complex situations. Partner violence in a loving relationship is definitely a confusing and complex situation. These questions express our need for a clear, straightforward story with a culprit because it tells us what to do in such circumstances. Finally, they are part of the cycle itself.

These three reasons make it very understandable that couples ask these questions. We take on the frustrating position of not answering them—at least not in a simple, causal way. So, we ask for a little stretch of our readers' minds. We do this not to frustrate you but because we don't want to pour extra oil on the fire that is the cycle."

"What happened to you?"

What follows is an attempt to address the foundation beneath these questions without fueling the cycle. There is a need to understand what is happening so you know what you can do in such a complex, overwhelming situation. We have already started this: in Chapter 3, we described how to understand and organize what happens between you. However, a piece of the puzzle remains. "What then about our wounds? The history we carry with us?" There is another wisdom in the question, "What is wrong with me, with you, and with us?"—namely, "How can we situate our *vulnerability* and limitations within this story?"

Jef: "To reflect on this meaningfully without escalating the situation, we choose to turn the questions around somewhat. In doing so, we follow Bruce Perry's example on the Oprah Winfrey's show (Perry & Winfrey, 2021) where he asks the wonderful question, 'What happened to you?' We can perfectly flip the questions 'What is wrong with you, me, and us?' into 'What happened to me? What happened to you? What happened to us?' This opens the door to a story that allows for both clarity and complexity."

Lieven: "So, beneath the cycle is another story—a story about what happened to each of us and to us as a couple. How did we go from being a 'powerhouse' to a 'fight club'? We have already described how outside pressures, repeated small events, or major life themes create tension that organizes itself between people in a certain way: the interaction cycle. In the struggle for connection, we end up in that particular, recurring loop. Underneath it all, of course, there may be life experiences that make you more sensitive to needing and losing the 'Finally!' So, escalating conflicts do not all result from interaction patterns where people's protection becomes their relational prison. This is the wisdom behind the question of what is wrong: there are indeed things you carry with you that make you *more sensitive to the loss of love*."

Stories of vulnerability

Think back to the phrase we quoted in question three: "Partner violence = ordinary conflicts × 10." Apparently, there is something that causes ordinary conflicts to be experienced at ten times their usual intensity, a kind of sensitivity that amplifies the intensity. This is about a vulnerability that humans acquire through life.

Jef: "Let me illustrate this with an example. Everyone feels some concern when a loved one does not come home at the expected time. Regardless of your life experiences, you can imagine waking up at 2 a.m. to find that your partner is not lying next to you, even though they would normally return from ping-pong practice, Pilates, or whatever activity by 11 p.m. It feels good to have the freedom to go out. It's reassuring to see your partner leave for a place they enjoy, with the peace of mind that you will see them again soon. When they don't come back, it affects us. 'Oh dear…' That feeling triggers fears and anxieties. People react differently: one might wait and try to push the anxiety away, while another sends a message or tries to call.

But something can happen that *intensifies* that reaction. Imagine losing a parent at a young age. I have a client who experienced this—she was 12 years old when her father, a dedicated athlete, went jogging one day and never returned. He died of a ruptured artery. This is not something you simply get over. That experience can suddenly strike you very hard in everyday situations. If this woman's partner is still not home at 2 a.m., her feelings will be very different. It's not just anxiety; it's pure panic racing through her veins. Her reaction matches that intensity. It's not just sending one message—it's nine texts in one minute; calling repeatedly; jumping into the car in pajamas; pacing at the entrance of the sports hall; then launching into a tirade once they are finally driving home together."

The question "Is something wrong with me or you?" is dangerous because it fuels the cycle and promotes a simplistic "one cause, one culprit" view that detracts from a complex reality. At the same time, this question reveals important life sensitivities that help us understand escalating conflicts. These sensitivities cause people to experience intense emotions in ordinary life events.

For those involved in fierce escalations, it certainly makes sense to ask, "What happened in your life that makes you particularly vulnerable to this or that behavior?" Such questions uncover a wealth of complex stories that, rather than blaming, open the door to understanding. Partner violence is primarily a circular dynamic involving two people. As we said before, the "partner" part is crucial. Beyond that, two individuals bring with them a history filled with all kinds of experiences that shape their shared narrative.

Jef: "To me, this feels like a *library of all the stories* life has taught people. I see clients in front of me—like the woman I mentioned. A wonderful young woman who lost her father far too soon and

> suddenly. Since then, she has been especially sensitive to loved ones who distance themselves from her. I also think of other stories from the library. An older man told me about the immense aggression he experienced growing up because of his father—a constant rain of accusations, blame, humiliation, and seeing his father beat his mother unconscious. This is a completely different story in the library. This man has carried so much anger, in a very destructive way. Now, when his wife expresses any criticism, or when there is tension between the children, tremendous stress floods him. His body tenses, and anxiety takes over. Even though his mind knows his father has long been dead, the same panic overwhelms him. He rushes out of the house as fast as he can. He is terrified: 'There is anger in my family. This makes me very nervous. I'm afraid I'll snap under this stress, and that would be awful because I swore I would never be like my dad.' So, he leaves. That reaction makes sense if you listen to his story. The trauma still lives in his body and is triggered by anger, criticism, and raised voices in the present. When he leaves, his wife often follows. She carries her own sensitivity to loneliness, having lost important people who were not there for her when she needed them.
>
> Put those two stories together, and the relational cycle begins again. It's the cocktail of what happens between people and what has happened to them in their lives that can trigger something as complex as partner violence."

The stories of those caught in escalating conflicts are diverse, yet a pattern emerges. They are deeply individual stories that can be grouped by a central theme: Were the relationships with those who cared for me—those I liked—safe? Was I seen by them? Did I belong? Was I important to them? Beneath these individual vulnerabilities runs a common thread: *attachment*.

Couple pain

In some cases, beneath the flare-ups of partner violence lies a vulnerability rooted in individual suffering or trauma. In such situations, the question "What happened to you, and what happened to me?" can be extremely helpful. In other cases, however, it is the couple's shared history—painful events that occurred within the relationship—that intensifies the negative interaction cycle. In these moments, questions like "What happened to us?" or "What happened to our relationship?" are often more relevant.

Lieven: "Sometimes things happen to us as a couple that create vulnerability or sensitivity within the relationship—a child dies, there's a bankruptcy, infidelity. We call this an *attachment injury*. In some instances, these painful events touch on earlier experiences in our lives, making them harder to process or endure. In other cases, events occur in the relationship that elicit overwhelming emotions, even if they're not connected to earlier life experiences. The event itself is profoundly painful.

This kind of *relational pain* can linger for a long time. That's really a different section in your library, Jef. I think of Davy and Kris, a gay couple I've seen for some time. Davy keeps returning to his partner's infidelity early in the relationship. Kris becomes desperate: 'I've told you—it's in the past! It's over!' But no matter what Kris says or does, he can't seem to ease Davy's anxiety. Infidelity, especially repeated infidelity, is a common attachment injury that many couples struggle to move beyond. These injuries can make even everyday conflicts instantly intense. For example, if Kris distances himself during an argument, Davy doesn't just think, 'He'll cool off and come back.' No—Davy is convinced Kris is going to see someone else, because of that unresolved relational pain.

Another couple I work with was affected by a very different issue: money. They had a lot of it—an extraordinary amount. Then, suddenly, the husband became entangled in lawsuits and was convicted of fraud. Overnight, the money was gone. The judgmental gaze of the outside world pierced the couple. The security they once shared crumbled. The wife lashed out: '*What did you do? How could you risk our safe world—the future of our children?*' The distrust and insecurity born in that moment still live on in their relationship, even years later. They haven't been able to repair that rupture."

Jef: "I immediately think of Stephan and Sandra, another couple I see. They faced professional struggles. Stephan had dreamed of owning his own woodworking business for years. Eventually, he quit his salaried job with a contractor and took the leap. Sandra believed in him. She supported his dream wholeheartedly and even joined the business to manage the administration—an area Stephan struggled with. At the time, this felt deeply connecting for them as a couple. Just as the business began to find its footing, the

COVID-19 crisis hit. Like many, they were unprepared. Financially, things were already tight, and this was the final blow. The dream collapsed. Their shared project disintegrated. The impact on their relationship was immense. They lost confidence in each other. They started pointing fingers. Again, their sense of security was shattered, and the familiar questions returned: *'Are you still there for me? Do you still love me? Am I still good enough for you?'*

So let's be clear: it's not only early childhood experiences that matter. Experiences shared as a couple can also create vulnerabilities."

In addition to individual vulnerability or early childhood trauma, we also consider the history of the couple. There is a kind of "library" that contains not only personal experiences but also *emotional wounds from past relationships*. For example, your current partner may not have been unfaithful, but you might have experienced infidelity with one or more previous partners. While this may not relate directly to your parents or your current partner, it can still intensify conflicts in your current relationship.

Lieven: "Especially today, with so many blended and reconstituted couples, these past experiences are incredibly important. How did your previous relationship end? For instance, were you suddenly abandoned without explanation? That kind of experience can leave someone more sensitive to emotional distance in a new relationship—even when the current partner is entirely trustworthy and has no idea where that distrust is coming from.

To be thorough, we should also acknowledge that these different histories often *converge*. Let's take your earlier example, Jef, of the couple who started a business together. In such cases, there is almost always one partner who dreams bigger and more boldly than the other. In this case, perhaps that's Stephan. Sandra is the more cautious partner, following along but with some anxiety. At first, things go well, and this fuels her admiration for the dreamer. But then a crisis hits. For Stephan and Sandra, it was an external event—COVID-19. Sometimes the crisis is internal—maybe the dreamer is careless with financial details. The debts begin to accumulate.

Sandra, being more cautious, starts to notice and becomes anxious. Something shifts. She becomes angry with herself for having followed the dream. That anger turns outward, and she slams on the brakes. Stephan, in turn, feels betrayed: 'What are you doing?

Things are already difficult, and now you're holding me back when I'm trying to fix the problem?' Beneath this dynamic in the present, shaped by the crisis they're facing as a couple, there are often deeper, earlier histories at play. For instance, how money, security, and desire were managed in childhood. Sandra may have grown up in poverty, which intensifies her anxiety and her impulse to hit the brakes. Stephan, on the other hand, may have grown up in an environment where he was never allowed to dream, where every expression of individuality was stifled. When you combine all of this, you have a volatile mix—one that doesn't need much to tip into conflict, or even violence."

Questions that close; questions that open

The way we ask questions like "What's wrong with you, me, or us?" can have very different effects. If we ask from a place of fear and emotional reactivity, such questions often reinforce and even intensify negative patterns. But if we ask from a desire to understand and a genuine curiosity about how to move forward, the effect changes entirely. Then the question might sound more like: "Hey, what happened to you that makes you so sensitive to what's going on between us? I want to understand. I want to understand you. Would you explain it to me?" Do you feel how different that is? It opens the door to a library of stories—personal narratives, shared couple histories, and each partner's individual relationship past.

Jef: "The tone in which we ask a question like, 'What's wrong with you, me, or us?' often carries an undertone of blame and can sound frightening. It can make you feel like something is fundamentally broken—that you, your partner, or the relationship is flawed or doesn't belong. It's only natural to want to protect yourself in response. You hide your vulnerable parts. You bury the core. Sometimes you even lose the words to describe what's going on. You start doing whatever you can to avoid feeling overwhelmed.

But when we shift the question toward curiosity—toward the stories that make us vulnerable—it opens the door to each other's inner world. We begin to welcome each other's history, the essence of who we are. In those moments, something remarkable happens: a *language for vulnerability* begins to emerge. That language has two parts. First, people begin to speak; their capacity to express themselves grows. And second, I notice that their ability to listen grows, too. Their ears become more attuned to a story that is now being told in a new way.

Conflict brings speed. It accelerates emotion, and in that rush, we often lose the ability to articulate what we feel. It's like trying to find the right book in a library while running. In that confusion, you protect yourself, and you become incomprehensible to the other. But the question 'What happened to you?' slows everything down. Suddenly, people are walking together in the library. They explore the shelves and find the book that speaks to their vulnerability. Watching that happen is always powerful. It doesn't just help people understand their conflict better—it helps them understand each other more deeply.

I see so many couples stuck in escalating conflict for years. But when they reach the point where they can ask together, 'What is happening to us? What's happening to you? This is what's happening to me. What have we lived through that makes us so vulnerable here?'—that becomes a *turning point*. Where they were once hurting each other, an opening is created for a deeper understanding of who they are today—in the world and in their relationship with each other."

Subtitles to the tough exterior

To move from sharing stories to resolving conflict, one crucial link is still missing. Many people already know large parts of each other's histories. They know, for instance, that their partner's father died when she was 12, or that his childhood was shaped by constant criticism. They may even recognize the emotional tone of that pain. In that sense, the stories themselves are not always new. What we're really looking for in retelling them is the connection to the *present*—to how that old pain is reawakened in the day-to-day experience of living and arguing together.

Jef: "If we return to the couple I mentioned at the beginning of this conversation, something shifts: the partner begins to understand that staying away after training triggers a deeply rooted fear of abandonment. Or the wife comes to realize that the loud, angry voices of their arguing children evoke in her husband the tension of anticipated aggression—and that her critical remarks cause him to shrink back, overwhelmed by the feeling of being a complete failure.

Before this insight, partners only see the surface of each other's behaviors: angry, persistent text messages when one is away for a while, or a partner who withdraws the moment things become challenging with the children. These behaviors are unpleasant, often provoke misunderstanding, and leave both feeling powerless. But when those behaviors are connected to the underlying emotional story, a completely different narrative emerges. 'Ah! So every time you send an angry text, it's because you're afraid of losing me?' That's what we call the *missing link*—the essential piece of the puzzle. It provides *subtitles*, making visible what was previously invisible. These subtitles help us recognize that old stories—traumas, fears, emotional patterns—still live in our bodies and are reactivated in the present moment. That connection is crucial. It enables couples to respond differently, *turning conflict into opportunities for learning rather than for rupture.*

Imagine combining these two perspectives into a conversation like this:

She: 'Every time I feel you're gone too long, my heart races. Every cell in my body screams, *He's leaving too. He won't come back. I'll be left alone again.* The thought of losing you sends me into such a panic that I can't do anything but reach out. So I call you—again and again—each text message angrier than the last.'

He: 'I don't want to leave you. I want nothing more than to be close to you. But when I see those angry messages, I feel like I can't say anything. I shut down. It's like I'm shrinking until I almost disappear. All I feel is that I've failed completely—that I'm a disappointment in your eyes. You don't say it directly, but in my mind, I hear the relentless, scathing words of my father. I can't silence them—they just get louder. I can only run from that feeling so I can breathe again. But in doing so, I end up running from you, too. And that just makes you even more afraid that I'll leave.'"

At the speed of conflict, we rarely find these words. In those moments, silence takes over and our bodies begin to speak for us. Her messages grow angrier. His distance increases. When they are finally back in the same space, it is no surprise that things escalate, sometimes even violently. But when time is taken afterward to *slow* things down and let these underlying stories come to the surface, violence is no longer necessary. The subtitles allow them to understand each other more deeply and feel more connected. She no longer feels abandoned. He begins to feel seen as capable and valued in her eyes. Then, even with their vulnerabilities and histories, this couple can move forward—together.

Making room for disabilities

Up to this point, we have deliberately avoided the question, "What is wrong?" At the same time, there are situations in which something truly is wrong—flaws, deficits, disabilities. It's a fine line, but consider a case where one partner has, for example, bipolar disorder. That's not something you recognize immediately. It may take several cycles of mania and depression before you conclude, "Something is wrong here," and seek help from a psychiatrist. In such cases, it can be helpful for the couple to begin with, "Something is wrong (with you)." What follows is a discussion of how to make room for disabilities in relationships, without reducing the entire dynamic of partner violence to a diagnosis.

Lieven: "You know, I have a hearing problem. It bothers me tremendously. Yesterday I was on a fan bus heading to the Ghelamco Arena to watch a football game with my granddaughter. The music was blasting. There was a woman who was already drunk before we even arrived, and she kept shouting instead of talking. Just noise everywhere. My granddaughter was saying something, and I had to ask her seven times to repeat it. It was incredibly frustrating—for both of us. Life includes disabilities. Violent couples also need to make space for these kinds of challenges, or what I sometimes call '*niggles*.' But this isn't a simple category. Take depression, for instance. It's a word that's often thrown around too casually. Yet clinical depression is real and must be taken seriously. It can have a profound impact on individuals and couples alike. And there are many such conditions—ADHD, autism spectrum disorder (ASD), or a brain injury following a car accident...."

We first consciously moved away from the search for simple, linear explanations—only to return to them, because ignoring this possibility can distort reality. It's still a very fine line. Consider a recent email we received: "Dear [therapist], my husband and I fight a lot, and sometimes it gets really out of hand. Can we come see you? I should add that I think my husband is a narcissist." At first glance, you might think, "This is a disability we need to take into account." But in couples therapy, it's often quickly apparent that such labels reveal more about the experience of a pursuing partner who has lost connection with a more withdrawn one. This is just one example of many—cases where what seems like a disability is actually a relational dynamic, or a reflection of one partner's personal history, or the couple's shared history. At the same time, there are conditions that cannot and should not be reduced to relational explanations.

Lieven: "I wrote about this in another book (Migerode, 2026): we're all put together a little crooked. Everyone is a bit 'dotty,' as we say. But some people are more skewed than others. How do you explain that difference? It's a hard distinction to make, and people are often too quick to reach for a diagnosis. Because it's a simple explanation—and, as we've said before, our brains like simple explanations.

Take bipolar disorder, for example. I know people with very intense emotional fluctuations who are not bipolar. But when those fluctuations reach a certain point, the diagnosis becomes a form of protection—a marker of something insurmountable. No matter what you do, the swings are there. You end up back in the pit, or back in the mania. When someone lives with that, we need to take it into account.

It's easy to say, 'My husband has ASD,' but sometimes in therapy you encounter someone whose way of communicating is genuinely different—so different that it's much harder to connect. That's when we must keep asking: where does the story of '*What happened to you, to me, or to us?*' end, and where does '*What's wrong with you, me, or us?*' begin?

And again, the answer has to do with attachment. In a secure relationship, there is room for *disabilities*. In that case, it's essential to know what's going on with each other, in order to deal with it. But in the insecure, reactive cycle of cause and effect, the search for 'what's wrong' is rarely helpful."

Couple > individual > disability

There is a meaningful sequence here. We always begin with the couple's relational story. We look for the interactional cycle, and only once we've been able to separate that from who the couple is do we ask whether there's a narrative of something that happened or a disability that is present. Much must be peeled away before we can thoughtfully assess whether there's an unavoidable reality that remains. All too often, however, we see the opposite reflex: beginning with the assumption of disability. This leaves little space for the people involved and for the relationship itself. Our approach is different: we begin with the couple, with the people in the couple. Only then do we consider whether a disability is present. If it is, we explore how to thoughtfully integrate that into their shared story. It is a slower path, but one that honors complexity and leaves room for love.

Jef: "Let's go back to your hearing loss, Lieven. Because you're getting older (and also, let's face it, because you've had too many people nagging around your ears), you've become more sensitive to certain sounds. This makes the question 'What's happening between us, and how do we deal with it together?' very important but only in the context of secure attachment.

Think of the many trainings we lead together. There are always lots of people, so it's noisy. Naturally, there are times when you ask someone to repeat themselves, or you avoid sitting in the middle of the group during breaks. If I responded with, 'What's wrong with you? Do something about it!' it would harm our collaboration. But if we together give that disability a place in our relationship, we can think through its consequences. For example, when someone at the back of the room makes a comment, I now instinctively repeat it for you. I know that I'm hearing something you may not. And when I forget, and you let me know you didn't catch it, I immediately understand. That safe foundation allows us to move together to the question, 'How do we integrate this between us?' It gives us space to acknowledge the disability without making you feel like something is wrong with you as a person.

I have a disability, too: I stutter. During our trainings, I sometimes say strange things without realizing it. The problem is that I block on certain words, but I can often feel it coming. Over the years, I've learned to prepare mental detours—alternative words I won't stumble over. That leads to unusual sentence structures or word choices. Fortunately, you hear this, Lieven. Sometimes you'll intervene and say, '*What you mean is…*' even when I haven't noticed. And that feels safe. I feel cared for. But if, in that moment, you laughed and said, '*What's wrong with you, man?*'—then we'd have a problem."

Disabilities exist. They can play an important role in the dynamics of partner violence. But when they're used as a starting point, they often become an added obstacle for couples already struggling to see and hear each other. When partners are given space to explore their interaction patterns and individual histories, a more constructive space emerges in which disabilities—if they are present—can be acknowledged and addressed together. This allows the couple to carry the weight of the disability as a duo, just as Lieven and Jef have learned to carry their own vulnerabilities together.

Conclusion: building a soft bed

Conflict and violence in relationships bring fear and urgency. They push us to seek a quick, simple way out—often by blaming and removing the guilty party. But this approach leaves little room for connection or for the couple as a whole. We hear this dynamic in the questions people ask: "What is wrong with you, with me, and with us?" These questions arise logically from the patterns people are caught in. Our role is to redirect them toward exploring what happened in each person's story and in the couple's shared story. One partner may be scarred by certain life events, while the other carries a sensitivity of their own—often invisible at first, sometimes even part of what initially attracts them. This sensitivity slowly seeps into the relationship, transforming what began as a calm interaction into one charged with frightening intensity. These underlying stories rarely guide behavior consciously; they inhabit people's bodies—in a tone of voice, a laugh, an absent gaze—and then suddenly the body reacts, overwhelmed by the conflict monster. The cycle moves from the individual to the relationship and back again. In the vulnerability that arises from this curiosity and exploration, people are more likely to meet each other with quiet acceptance. Possible disabilities or vulnerabilities that emerge then find a soft bed on which to land. Within this bed, the couple can find space to carry the disability together, making it manageable.

The art of time and the choice of closeness—this is our wish for everyone reading this book. It means daring to slow down and truly listen to one another in the moments when space allows it. Can you feel the beauty of what can happen then? At the same time, you may become aware of how challenging this is. To know and show yourself in this way demands much from both the individual and the relationship. This brings us seamlessly to the next challenge: the courage to look these vulnerable parts in the eye, let alone to speak about them. Doing so requires overcoming a new hurdle—shame. We will take this up in the next chapter, where we explore what makes it so difficult to talk about these intense, intimate layers of who we are, both separately and together.

Reflect and relate

Take a moment to pause and connect these ideas to your own experience.

These questions are not about finding blame, but about slowing down to explore how your life story and your shared story as a couple might influence what happens between you.

1. When you think of moments when you get stuck in conflict, what do you notice that makes these moments especially painful or difficult for you?

2. What has happened in your life that may make you extra sensitive when your partner comes very close/when they seem very far away (delete what doesn't apply for you)?

3. Have you or your partner been wounded in earlier relationships in ways that make the loss of connection in this relationship feel more intense?

4. Imagine saying to your partner (and delete what doesn't apply):

5. "When we argue and I feel not good enough / all alone, I tend to withdraw / pursue. Sometimes I react even more strongly—it can turn into anger or aggression—because something inside me gets touched. Life made me extra sensitive to closeness / distance."

6. How would it feel to say this out loud?

7. How might it change your conflicts if you both shared what life has taught you about closeness, distance, and fear of loss?

References

Migerode, L. (2016). *Ik zie u graag. Hoe blijf je gelukkig in je relatie.* Lannoo.

Perry, B., & Winfrey, O. (2021). *What happened to you? - Conversations on trauma, resilience and healing.* Spectrum.

5
WHY IS IT SO HARD TO TALK ABOUT THIS?

Talking about moments when things get out of hand is not easy. It feels very vulnerable to reveal to others how difficult things really are and to share some of the complex feelings that race through you in those situations. You don't know how someone will react if you say you threw a vase at your partner's head. You don't know how they will look at you when you tell them the hole in the door is from your fist, which missed your wife's jaw by inches. You don't know if you will still be welcome when you admit the bruise isn't from falling down the stairs, but from being pushed—and that despite all this, you still love each other deeply. Who will understand that? If I struggle to understand it myself, how can I explain it to others?

"They're going to think I'm weak, reprehensible. They'll say I married a monster and that we should separate. They'll say I'm crazy. They'll say I brought it on myself." Sharing such painful stories takes immense courage and trust, and that trust is often already compromised among people caught in escalating conflicts. Society's perception of partner violence often fuels overwhelming shame. That image leaves little confidence that you will be met with acceptance for your suffering or for your own story.

It's not only speaking outwardly that triggers shame. Showing yourself fully to your partner is daunting enough. Letting down your guard to say

DOI: 10.4324/9781003683582-6

how small and vulnerable you feel, how ashamed you are of your outburst, how afraid you are of losing control again, how deeply you fear losing him or her—again—damages trust in the other's response.

So, there are many reasons to remain silent and hide. Yet, escalating conflicts and the intense emotions they bring can be so overwhelming that staying alone with them feels unbearable. In this chapter, we reflect on this paradox that traps so many people.

The many obstacles in speaking

A relationship can be so important, and the feelings of powerlessness and wordlessness so great, that aggression, either seeking closeness or pushing away, arises. This aggression tries to communicate something that cannot be expressed in any other way. This dynamic happens between people as part of the conflict cycle. Additionally, people sometimes feel powerless after the flood of emotions has passed because they long to talk about it but find their shame and fear too great to share with each other or with others around them.

When we consider why it is so difficult to talk about these issues, we ask two related but distinct questions: First, "Why is it so hard to talk about this with others?" and second, "Why is it so hard to talk to each other?" Both involve shame, but different types or expressions of shame.

Lieven: "I just had a ninety-minute conversation with a new couple. They cannot talk about the conflicts they frequently have. Because the wife doesn't express what bothers her clearly, she gets loud and uses threatening words. These words intimidate her husband so much that he becomes silent, which only causes her to grow louder, using words like 'always' and 'never.' He becomes even more silent and distant. They have been trapped in this cycle for 20 years. I asked, 'These problems have lasted 20 years. What have you tried to do about them?' She said, 'I wish we could talk about it, but we can't. Every time we try, we immediately fall back into the same dynamic.' For this couple, *the cycle* itself prevents real conversation. Instead of a dialogue between two people, it becomes a confrontation between two defenses. Speaking, especially how they speak, creates fear in both: 'What I want to share doesn't matter to him. He's not there for me,' and 'Whatever I say won't be good for her, so I won't start.' Naturally, he increasingly avoids talking, and she only brings concerns forward more aggressively. Genuine conversation becomes impossible."

Jef: "There are indeed two layers: the inability to speak as part of the cycle, which differs from the difficulty of speaking about it with others—family, friends, or counselors. If we focus on speaking to others, it's striking that people receive a *double message*. On one hand, there is the persistent assumption that talking about it is the solution. Almost every campaign about partner violence says: 'Talk about it! Don't stay alone with your story.' On the other hand, most messages emphasize that partner violence is dangerous and forbidden. So, if you struggle with this yourself, you are stuck: violence is forbidden—it's not allowed—but talk about it and don't stay alone. If talking is supposed to be the solution, it's important to acknowledge this impossibility and give it space."

The situation in which the negative interaction cycle prevents real conversation was described extensively in previous chapters. The intense fear on both sides makes it logical to avoid expressing vulnerability, to avoid showing oneself without protective layers—and paradoxically, that very protection leads to escalating conflict. Furthermore, we often observe in practice that when couples step out of escalations and experience a moment of calm, they want to convey something meaningful about what happened, but this becomes frightening in a new way. This seems to be when *shame* often appears: "If I show my partner how scared or vulnerable I am, they won't like me anymore."

Lieven: "On the one hand, people fear that if they finally talk about it, the cycle will start again. Once things are calm, they want to avoid at all costs losing control again. Especially with violence, there is fear that discussing the blows or boundary violations will trigger a new cycle. 'If I tell her how scared I've been since she pushed me down the stairs, she won't see me as a man, and things will only get worse.' Or, 'If I tell him how deeply hurt I am since he insisted on sex when I wasn't feeling well, he'll just get angry.'

On the other hand, shame prevents us from revealing the vulnerability beneath the argument, both to each other and to others. In either case, it is the eyes of the other that make us hide. The fear of rejection and being judged negatively combines with our own fear of exposing our 'dirty laundry.' Everyone around us condemns it, and we do too. *So, both internally and externally, there is a barrier to speaking and showing.*"

Is it safe to speak to the environment?

When we work with couples in conflict, we always say, "What you are suffering from is complex and layered. It has a lot to do with love and the powerlessness that can arise from that, and you are welcome to bring your whole story." Then we begin working with those couples. They start revealing the cycle, and together we try to construct a logical narrative. If we sense that the intensity of the interaction cycle is high, at some point, we ask, "Does it ever get out of hand?" At that moment, hesitation almost always appears in the therapy room. The threshold for speaking up is palpable. Couples rarely cross it easily.

Jef: "Just last week, it happened again. Levi and Ella are a young couple I've been working with for some time. When I asked whether things ever get out of hand when they're caught in the cycle, there was a brief moment of silence. They made quick eye contact—just a moment of shared stillness. What emerged was hesitation, a palpable mix of panic and ambivalence: *Are we going to talk about this? Should we talk about this?*

It was as if, in that fleeting glance—so rare for them, given how often they struggle to attune to one another—they made a joint risk assessment: *Is it safe, here and now, to reveal this vulnerable and hurt part of ourselves?* I could really feel them scanning me for the answer.

Two forces were at play: one urging them to speak, the other holding them back, unsure of the consequences. They risked hearing, yet again, that things aren't okay—that *they* aren't okay, that their partner isn't okay, and that their relationship isn't okay.

When I saw that hesitant, searching look on their faces, I slowed down and made space for it—*before* they answered the question. I said, 'It doesn't seem easy to answer. Your glance at each other looked like you were trying to figure out if it's safe to talk about this. Talking about this carries risk. Do you feel that?'

That acknowledgment created room to explore their hesitation and, at the same time, lowered the threshold for talking about the violence. This kind of moment doesn't happen everywhere. In fact, Levi and Ella told me they had seen another therapist before—who ended the therapy when they disclosed this part of their relationship.

Such a shame, because we ended up having a very meaningful conversation that brought a lot of relief to both of them. Unfortunately, it wasn't the first time I'd heard that couples had to stop seeing their therapist after opening up about the violence between them."

Lieven: "What strikes me about Levi and Ella's story is how much they work *together* in the moment when you, as a therapist, ask whether things sometimes spiral out of control—despite the fact that, in other moments, they're so lost in escalation and violence. In that brief look they shared, they made a joint decision: Are we going to take the leap? Maybe with Jef…

And even when they do take that leap, they remain afraid as they speak.

I think it's important to make a crucial distinction when we talk about the importance of speaking. It might sound as though speaking is the solution. For us, it's not. Speaking is, however, a necessary step toward change. It creates space for people to step into a different interaction pattern. Speaking is a step. Just like confronting or facing something is a step.

But speaking also carries risk. It can halt therapy, even when you're asking for help with your relationship. It can lead to questions about the children, or bring external scrutiny. So, speaking is both necessary and dangerous.

That's why I want to stress to people: speaking up isn't always safe. Don't speak to just anyone. As a couple, take the space to sense where it is safe. What Levi and Ella did makes perfect sense. They checked in with each other: 'Do we both want this?' and 'Do we want to do this with Jef? Is it safe with him?' Anyone struggling with partner violence has likely already faced the choice of whether to talk about it—or has experienced opening up and being warmly received, only to later encounter a fearful or judgmental response."

When we speak, what will the environment do?

In that moment of eye contact between a couple—when they decide whether or not to speak up—we can sense Ella and Levi's hesitation. There are at least three major reasons for this.

The first is the fear: "What will happen to us if we talk about this? Will it spiral out of control and drag us back into the cycle again?" The second is: "How will others see us if we reveal this?" This is where shame often silences people. We'll explore that more deeply later in this chapter. And finally: "What will be expected of us if we admit that partner violence is happening? What will the consequences be?"

Particularly in the second and third reasons, notice how powerfully we are influenced by how we perceive ourselves through the eyes of others. Our relationships are shaped not only by how we experience them privately but also by how we present them—and how they are perceived—publicly. Are we a good couple or a bad one?

Jef: "Let's take a closer look at that last question, '*What will happen next?*', through the story of Levi and Ella. After yet another argument, Levi walks out and goes to his parents. Or Ella meets a close friend and confides that things have really gone too far with Levi: '*We were really shouting. We said such cruel things to each other. It escalated and eventually turned physical.*'

Whether it's Levi or Ella talking, those they confide in, especially loved ones, often feel compelled to act. There's something about this topic that makes people speed up and take a stand. It's logical, even compassionate. They care about Levi and Ella and want the violence to stop. But Levi and Ella may not experience that reaction as helpful. My guess is that what they most need is simply a space to talk about what's happening to them."

Lieven: "*So the third risk of speaking out is this: the listener—the surrounding environment—may not want to talk*. They may want to act. And in that moment, speech is lost.

You didn't want action; you wanted dialogue. You were hoping to say: 'Do you understand me? Can you see how hard this is? Can we think it through together? Can I fall apart for a moment? Can I voice my thoughts out loud before someone tells me what to do?' That longing is so understandable. When we see someone we care about suffering, we instinctively want to fix it. We don't want them to hurt. So we act, act, act. Or we push the suffering person to act:

> *'You can't stay with someone like that. There's only one solution: break up!'*
> *'Make him go to aggression therapy!'*
> *'Give her an ultimatum: either she gives you more freedom, or it's over.'*

> *'You need to stop drinking. That's when things go wrong.'*
> *'You have to set firmer boundaries.'*
> *'Let me tell you how she should handle this. She's just expecting too much. Give me five minutes with her and she'll act differently.'*
> *'Losing control like that isn't normal. You can't do that.'*
> *'Think of the children. Just fix it and move on—this fighting will scar them for life.'"*

When someone you care about is caught in a painful, escalating conflict with their partner, it's deeply distressing to witness. Hearing about the violence or witnessing the aftermath often stirs a sense of outrage. Naturally, this prompts an urge to stop it. But if you look closely at that list of reactions, you might also feel something else—something from the other side of the story. When a couple begins to reveal the violence in their relationship, there's a sudden rush of advice, of demands for action, of pressure. The urgency and intensity of that pressure, while well-meaning, often aren't helpful. In fact, the couple is already living under enormous pressure. Their relationship is already speeding out of control. They're stuck. They're exhausted. They feel trapped. So when they finally reach out—looking for peace, for gentleness—what they often collide with is a tidal wave of reaction and judgment from someone they love.

What they truly need is delay and space. How much space do we, as their community, give them to catch their breath? To reflect on what's happening? To decide, for themselves, what they want to do? To what extent do we see the depth of their struggle—and recognize the efforts they are already making to deal with it?"

Lovingly slowing down

We want to offer something to those who have a daughter, cousin, best friend, mother, neighbor, or colleague who comes to them with a story like this. When someone shares such an experience with you, it means they trust you. In that moment, all they are asking is: "Please, listen to me." They are not expecting you to do anything.

Lieven: "Of course, it's easy for us to say that. So I try to make it more concrete. Imagine your 11-year-old son comes home and says, 'I'm being bullied.' A typical response might be that Dad rushes to school and scolds the other child. But that's not what the son wanted. Now the situation might be even harder for him. What he really needed was for Dad to say, 'Oh no, buddy, that's awful. Are you okay? What do you want to do about it? Can I help you?' When we love someone, the protective, caring reflex is natural. The urge to take action is an expression of love. We don't want to dismiss that. The instinct to help is a good thing. But we hope to offer something that helps people recognize this reflex and pause it—so that they can first create space for the story to be told. When people feel that space, it opens up the freedom to make their own decisions about how to respond."

Jef: "The father in that story sympathizes with his son and understandably wants to act. He might even feel like shaking the bully himself. Or a mother might say, 'You can't deal with this alone. You have to tell the teacher tomorrow. And if you don't, I will.' Others might say, 'If someone hits you, hit them back—then they'll leave you alone,' or, 'The best fight is one you avoid. Just run when they come.' There's an endless stream of advice and reactions when suffering and violence are revealed. But that instinct to act needs to be tempered because something else is often needed, especially when someone is hurting and stuck.

Think about the times your child has taken a bad fall. Your daughter bangs her head on the edge of the table and starts bleeding. Yes, something might need to be done: stitches, cleaning the wound, a bandage. But first, what she needs is to come to you. To be held and reassured: 'Come here, sweetie. That must have scared you. *I'm right here.* It's going to be okay.' Only then comes the explanation: 'You fell pretty hard. That happens. Let's take a look. It's bleeding a lot, but we'll take care of it.' There's something in that tone—gentle, calming—that tells her she doesn't need to be afraid, and she's not alone."

These moments return us to the core attachment questions: *If I fall and get hurt, is someone there for me? If I tell you about a difficult situation I've gotten into, do I still belong? Am I still good enough for you?*

When we, as a community, react too quickly, we risk unintentionally answering those questions with a "no." As described earlier, much of the anger and aggression we see stems from the loss of that secure connection: "I'm not good enough for her." "He doesn't care about me." "We just don't belong together." In those moments of disconnection, someone might reach out to someone else. But if that person immediately springs into action, that negative response is reinforced: Again, not good enough. Again, not important. Again, not belonging. We believe that, despite our best intentions, we sometimes leave people alone in their pain. And when someone repeatedly experiences that kind of response—from loved ones or society—it's no wonder they lose confidence and stop speaking about it. Logically, this increases the internal tension and thus increases the chance for an escalation between the partners.

During or after the escalation?

What we've described so far is the situation where someone tries to talk about what happened after the fact. But what if we are present during the conflict? If you're in the middle of a situation where a couple is escalating—if you're in the action—it does make sense to act. Think again of children: if your two kids are fighting, you separate them. That's not the time for quiet reflection. Just like when one of them runs into the street—you act. Immediate safety comes first. So, if the couple is actively caught in a conflict, it's appropriate to follow your instinct to intervene. If you see your brother and his partner caught in an intense argument, and you're there, and it feels right to step in, it may help to pull someone aside, offer calm, and see what can be done to defuse the tension.

But that is very different from what's needed *after* the conflict when your brother later finds the courage to talk to you. If you jump in then with advice and directives, there's a good chance he won't bring it up again. And if he finds the strength to talk about it with his partner in therapy, only to be told, "As long as there's violence, I can't help you—this therapy has to stop," he might retreat for good. That ends the conversation. The space for speaking closes, and the couple is left alone with their pain.

Lieven: "What's most tragic about this is that we, as a society, create a kind of pressure cooker. People are in serious trouble and they know it, but they feel pressure to keep it to themselves. And yet, every one of us knows that when we're stressed—about anything—we need to talk about it. It's such a relief to share your thoughts with someone. It's vital not to be left alone in it.

That's why it's so important that our children, for example, can talk to someone—a godparent, a grandparent, or a friend—when they're angry with us. They can speak more freely to someone else, and that helps them stay connected to us as well. Maybe, eventually, they'll even come talk to us directly.

Our social reflex to take immediate action when someone discloses partner violence is completely understandable. But by reacting that way, we often push people further into a place where the action feels forced—and that's exactly what we hope to avoid. What we really want is for them to find another way to engage with the situation. And the beginning of that is talking. So, for couples or individuals who still feel able to talk to someone, we want to encourage them to seek out those who are safe enough to hear them say: 'I want to tell you something. But you don't need to do anything about it.'"

The complexity of speaking

It is a natural reaction to feel shocked when someone starts talking about escalation or violence. You don't want your son to be in a relationship where he and his partner hit each other. You don't want your niece to be shouted at during arguments until she feels worthless. You don't want the kind neighbor boy to have his face scratched open by a partner who is drunk and angry. Hearing or witnessing this evokes an immediate reflex of concern. Unfortunately, the response from listeners is often not as helpful as intended. That's one side of the story. But the story of partner violence is layered—full of different perspectives, experiences, and truths. What happens when all those elements collide? Let's reflect further on this complexity.

Jef: "No one can illustrate this better than people who live through it. I think of Anne. Whenever things escalated in her relationship with Cathy, she would go to her mother. Anne loves Cathy deeply. Cathy's family has struggled with her coming out as a lesbian and has responded with rejection. This weighs heavily on Cathy, and she finds it incredibly hard to cope. She becomes withdrawn. She stops going to work, avoids friends, takes less care of herself… she loses her zest for life. She takes medication—sometimes too much. Anne finds it painful to watch the strong, proud woman she fell in love with disappear. What began as support and understanding has slowly turned into exhaustion and despair. The more Anne tries to 'save' her wife, the more Cathy seems to fade. Cathy feels even more unworthy with every expression of concern: 'My family sees me as shameful, and now my wife sees me as a weak failure too. I'm just a burden to everyone.' They're stuck.

Eventually, things started to escalate physically. Anne violently shook Cathy after yet another day of her not leaving the sofa. Cathy, startled, pushed Anne away instinctively. Anne fell and bruised her arm. A few weeks later, another violent incident occurred. More recently, these episodes have become increasingly frequent. Sometimes Cathy shuts down completely; other times, she fights back or even loses control. In these moments, Anne breaks her silence and turns to her mother, overwhelmed. She tells her, 'Life with Cathy is unbearable. She's crazy. Look what she did!'

It is completely understandable. Anne tells the story from her point of view, after being alone with it for so long. She's seeking understanding. But in doing so, she shares only the painful, one-sided version. Her mother responds: *'It's time for you to leave Cathy. She's destroying you. She's no longer welcome here.'* At first, Anne feels relief: *'At least my mom sees how hard this is for me.'* But once she's back home and things have calmed down, she feels even more trapped. Cathy is already estranged from her own family, and now she's unwelcome in Anne's family as well. Cathy retreats further into isolation, and Anne's despair deepens."

It makes sense that people confide in family or friends during moments of acute pain—and in doing so, share only one side of the violence. There are often no words yet for the other side: that they still love their partner, and that the other person has their own story and perspective. At the same time, this makes it very difficult for the listener to stay calm and keep an open mind about the relationship.

Lieven: "Just as a couple finds it difficult to truly hear each other when tensions are high and they're caught in the cycle and only manage to do so more effectively once things have calmed down, it's similarly hard for the surrounding environment to remain neutral or inactive when the tension is intense and the violence still palpable. Calm brings perspective—for both the couple and those around them. Nuance and circularity become far more visible and tangible when the situation is no longer inflamed.

In the heat of conflict, we sometimes need to roar—like a child who cries out after a fall. The cry is sharp with fear and pain, even though the actual harm is often minimal. But that child still needs comfort in that moment of panic. Providing that care requires something different from the support needed later, once the fear has subsided. This metaphor extends to partner violence. People need care while they are still 'roaring'—frightened and overwhelmed. At the same time, the care required afterward is also essential, and it is of a different nature."

Talking about partner violence is increasingly proving to be a path filled with obstacles. When couples attempt to discuss it, they inevitably touch on deeply vulnerable themes—topics they often can't risk addressing vulnerably, which is understandable given their history of conflict. Yet, when these issues are shrouded in layers of self-protection, they can become fuel for new escalations. Trying to discuss them with others carries further risks. One might be met with condemnation or pressured into drastic action at a time when what is actually needed is rest, reflection, and space to slow down. Who would dare to take such a dangerous step? Only the naive, the reckless—or the truly courageous.

The courage to face shame

Speaking about partner violence also brings up another critical dimension we've touched on before: shame. It takes immense courage to talk about violence because doing so means admitting that you've done something, or are trapped in something, that you know isn't right, and that others likely disapprove of as well. It's terrifying to speak out when you're already burdened by internal condemnation. Shame signals that our moral compass is intact. Most of the people we speak with already believe that violence is unacceptable; they've internalized that social and moral value. It takes tremendous bravery to expose the ugliness and complexity of escalating conflicts.

Jef: "To admit that you've humiliated your partner, attacked them at their most vulnerable points knowing it would hurt, stomped on them, or squeezed their throat—even whether this was done alone or reciprocally, whether the other responds or not, whether the listener truly hears or not—there is always that fear: *'Now we don't belong anymore.'* Shame is an emotion that helps us stay connected to our group. It signals what is and isn't acceptable. When we think about aggression in our society, the dominant message is clear: aggression in relationships is unacceptable, and such relationships cannot be loving. To speak about this exposes you to the stigma that you're not okay, that you don't belong, and that love isn't possible in your relationship. And in that moment, the part of you that is trying to do right and that is fighting for love becomes invisible. The longing to belong keeps many people silent—or at least hesitant to speak."

Lieven: "Again, this is a strange and painful process. Our internal condemnation of violence often compels us to remain silent for as long as we can. But that silence competes with the longing not to be alone in the experience. If we eventually reveal the violence in the hope of being cared for, seen, and understood—and are instead met with an embarrassed glance that says, 'That shouldn't happen'—we are thrown back on ourselves. In doing so, society only deepens the shame that was already there from the beginning."

An unbearable field of tension

People who experience partner violence firsthand often find themselves trapped in a painful contradiction. On one hand, there is the deep desire to speak out: "I want to say it so that I am no longer alone in this suffering. I want to feel seen and know that I still belong." On the other hand, there is a pervasive fear and conviction that revealing the violence will result in rejection—that they will no longer belong. Tragically, this fear is frequently reinforced by the very reactions they encounter when they do speak up. This dilemma applies both to conversations with others and to attempts to speak with their partner. What an impossible position this creates. And what a profound tension it carries. We have already described how this plays out in interactions with others. Let us now take a moment to consider the same tension within the context of communicating with one's partner.

Lieven: "Let me offer a very ordinary comparison. Imagine you're in a performance review with your boss and you accidentally pass gas. You don't need your supervisor to tell you that it's inappropriate in that context—you feel it yourself. Your embarrassment likely shows in the blush on your cheeks. We all know that tension: the anxiety about the reaction that might follow, and the instinct to withdraw from contact afterward. That kind of tension applies not just to social interactions but also within intimate relationships. It's incredibly difficult to tell your partner what you really feel underneath all your behaviors."

Speaking about the feelings that lie beneath a rough or reactive exterior requires time, patience, and—as we noted earlier—a great deal of courage. But that courage is often blocked by shame: "If I show this hurt part of myself, she won't like me anymore. She knows me as strong, calm, and reliable. If I reveal how small I feel inside, how could I possibly still be good enough for her?" Or, "If he sees how broken I am, I won't be attractive to him. He'll leave me." *These inner narratives, these "subtitles," can offer insight, but voicing them is incredibly stressful.* After carrying this pain alone for so long, not knowing how the other person will respond, the fear of rejection can be overwhelming. The risk of not being understood when exposing one's pain can make silence feel like the only safe option.

Jef: "Let me relate this to the couple I mentioned earlier. When Cathy feels like a total failure in the eyes of her family, her in-laws, and her partner—when she sees that she's barely managing, contributing little, and everything is falling on Anne's shoulders—she begins to think, 'I'm not doing anything right. I'm failing completely. I'm not worthy of Anne. She'll definitely leave me.'

Revealing that vulnerability to Anne stirs up immense shame. Cathy already feels deep shame about who she is as a daughter, an employee, a partner—and who she believes she should be. She fears that if she opens up to Anne, Anne might confirm her worst fear: 'Yes, you really do fall short. You're not enough.' That potential confirmation, layered on top of the intense shame already screaming inside her, is unbearable. She's terrified that sharing these feelings would mark the end of the relationship. So Cathy stays silent. It feels like the only option. But for Anne, that silence is excruciating: 'There's already so much I have to do on my own, and now you don't even want to talk to me. You won't share anything about how you feel… so I really am alone. Clearly, I don't matter to her.'"

Letting go of protection

It should be clear that it takes immense courage to reveal something vulnerable about yourself, especially when it risks confirming your deepest fears. In the midst of that pain, it often feels more bearable to remain alone with the harsh image you hold of yourself than to risk seeing that same image reflected in the eyes of others. And yet, if you were to show it, the outcome might not be as terrible as feared. Someone might still look at you with love—or even love you more than before. But it could also go the other way. You might see disdain, disappointment, or rejection, and that possibility evokes a fear so intense that it leads to self-protection: shame steps in. *Shame keeps us isolated with our worst self-perceptions, and at the same time shields us from the gaze and ears of others.*

Jef: "Let's return to Cathy and Anne. As Anne sees Cathy slipping away, she increasingly wonders, 'Why can't she get out of bed for me? Why does that chair seem more inviting than I am? I care about her so much, but all my care seems to be sliding off her.' Anne learned to care at a young age. Her father never regained joy in life after his business failed. As a child, she tried constantly to lift his spirits by getting good grades, excelling at basketball, and always showing up with a smile. Sometimes he smiled back, but his eyes never lit up again. Over time, Anne internalized a painful belief: 'I've spent my whole life caring for others, and it never seems to make a difference. What do I really mean to anyone?' So when Cathy withdraws, Anne begins to think, 'If she loved me, if I really mattered to her—if she could feel what I do for her—she'd be glad to see me. She'd want to go out with me.' But Anne doesn't dare speak those thoughts aloud. She fears that Cathy will confirm her worst suspicion: that her care truly doesn't matter, that she's not important. That fear is so distressing that she shifts into action. She starts saying things like, 'If you would just try a little harder, if you'd focus on the positives, it wouldn't be so terrible to come home here.' Like Cathy, Anne also begins to act rather than speak. 'See a therapist. Find a new job. Go for a walk—it would help you.' Her actions are driven by a desire to save her partner and their relationship but also to manage the anxiety beneath the surface. Anne fears that Cathy doesn't care about her, but she also fears the violence. She's afraid of losing control, afraid of Cathy's reactions, and worried things could escalate further. She's terrified that speaking up could provoke another violent episode. But we know from experience how these cycles work: the more Anne pushes, the more Cathy feels inadequate; the more Cathy withdraws, the greater the distance between them—and the more likely another incident of violence becomes."

Our experience tells us that Cathy and Anne would benefit greatly if someone could help them *talk* about their fears and vulnerabilities directly, *without the protection of defensive behaviors or the interference of action-driven responses.* In relationships where affection still exists, vulnerability often draws people closer. When we show the tender, hidden parts of ourselves, our partners are more likely to look at us with softer eyes.

Jef: "There's a good chance Anne would hear something like, 'But love, you have no idea how important you are to me. Your love is what keeps me going. Without it, I don't think I'd even be here. It's because I love you so much that I'm too ashamed to get out of that chair.'

And if they stayed with that moment, Cathy might say, 'I can't imagine ever being a good partner to you again. I do so little, and you give so much.' In response, Anne might say anything but what Cathy fears: 'I'm so glad you told me that. It's such a relief that you're not pushing me away because that's exactly what I've been afraid of. Now I can hear what's really going on inside you. When you show me that, I feel special to you again. I feel like your partner.' And just like that, something entirely different can happen: a connection begins to emerge, free of the obstacles that were keeping them apart."

Lieven: "If we ask what can help people break free from this cycle and overcome the mountain of shame, the answer lies in encouragement—encouragement to speak, despite the fear. And in that effort, we support every reader of this book. The internal image of being worthless, not good enough, unimportant to your partner, or not belonging—that is a devastating thing to carry. It makes it frightening to show your true self. But in hiding, you miss out on the *warm, tender gaze* that might meet you when you let go of your defenses and reveal yourself to someone who loves you. Through conversation, another way of relating can open up—a way that no longer needs silence, blame, substance use, or aggression to express what remained unsaid."

We've moved from the shame of speaking about violence with others and with one's partner to the shame of speaking about what sometimes *drives* the violence: the vulnerable and overwhelming feelings of not belonging, not being enough, or not being able to care well for someone you love deeply. There is a profound tension at the thought of speaking about these feelings but also a deep relief when they are finally expressed, and your partner doesn't get angry or walk away. In that moment, the terrifying image you had of yourself turns out not to live in your partner's eyes. And most importantly, you are no longer alone.

A deepening of shame

We've addressed the topic of shame several times already. It's a complex emotion, so it warrants further exploration. Nathanson developed a "compass of shame" that outlines four typical action tendencies resulting from this emotion: withdrawal, avoidance, attacking the self, and attacking others. These tendencies are frequently observed in cases of partner violence. Understanding the role of shame can provide deeper insight into such behaviors.

Lieven: "When you feel shame, you might put *yourself down*—'I'm worthless. I'm not okay. I can't do anything right.' These are depressive traits, which are quite evident in Cathy's case. A second response is to *blame* or attack the other person or the world, either verbally or physically—this is something we see in Anne. Then there's the urge to disappear, to want the ground to swallow you whole. This manifests in withdrawal and *isolation*, which Cathy also experiences. Finally, there's *avoidance*. While this may look like withdrawal, it's different. Rather than falling silent, the person becomes active—engaging in behaviors that help them avoid feeling shame. Addiction is a well-known example, but so is deliberately steering clear of anything that might trigger shame. People may throw themselves into activities simply to avoid feeling the emotion.

One person can exhibit several—or even all—of these action tendencies. Shame makes us leap in every direction to avoid the risk of being exposed. It whispers that such exposure would be unbearable."

Shame is a slippery emotion. It sparks behaviors that often reinforce the very cycle it stems from. When Cathy and Anne get caught in this cycle and aggression emerges, they start to feel, "This isn't okay. I don't want this. What we're doing isn't right. I'm going too far. If others saw this…." That moment brings them back to shame—fueling the cycle anew and making it even harder to speak. What started as a challenge becomes difficult, then extremely difficult, and eventually feels like an unscalable mountain.

The difficult task of supporters

Let us now return to the environment—those who are close to individuals experiencing partner violence. Consider Anne's mother or Cathy's best friend. They occupy a painful position: they hear the stories but cannot intervene directly. We've already mentioned that immediate action or advice isn't always helpful. So what can be done to support a couple burdened with such complex narratives and emotions?

Lieven: "When your daughter or best friend suddenly shows up at your door shaken, talking about a recent beating between her and her partner, of course you are shocked. This is an intense story. Naturally, you want to do everything possible to stop that suffering. If I may offer a roadmap: start at the beginning. Feel free to look for a wound that needs care. Of course, you may do that. If you want to do more, ask her, 'Is there anything I can do?' Sometimes she will say she needs shelter for a while—a bed for the night until things cool down. In most cases, the answer will be: 'Yes, listen and hold me tight. Don't walk away. Don't look at me differently when I tell you this. Don't stop liking me.' See the courage of Anne and Cathy, see the trust they place in you, and know they need your presence and reassurance to find the strength to speak differently to their partner. The calmer they tell you this, the easier it will be to listen and help them shape their own course of action.

It is wonderful that Anne and Cathy can come to you to cry out, vent, or reflect afterward. Give them space and time for their story and to find a new way to communicate. Let them feel how much you care so they don't remain alone and isolated with this experience. You may not realize how important your role as a listener and supporter can be."

Jef: "It is to be hoped that all the Cathys and Annes of the world can turn to such people—people with whom they can curse, cry, and be openly angry, sad, and scared after being hit or after giving physical or emotional blows, or a combination of both. I also hope that Cathy and Anne feel encouraged to speak honestly both with each other and with those who witnessed them when they were overwhelmed and vented in an unsubtle way a few days later, once the storm has passed. For anyone caught in escalating fights, a second conversation can reveal another side of the story: that they recognize their own part, feel ashamed, still care about the other person, want to find a solution together, or are considering ending the relationship but know it's a difficult decision they cannot make abruptly.

I learned from another client that I am asking something very difficult here. She is a woman I see for individual therapy. Her husband has crossed her sexual boundaries several times. They took breaks repeatedly. When he went too far, she left the house and stayed with friends. Her friends heard the stories of sexual assault. Together, they called a lawyer to start divorce proceedings and helped her retrieve her belongings. Yet, when she returned home after a week, she did not dare face her friends and avoided all contact—until things went wrong again. She said, 'If I told them how much I still like him, they would literally think I'm crazy. So, I no longer send messages or suggest meeting up.' From her, I learned how incredibly difficult it is to overcome the mountain of shame before the people you love. It's very hard, but if those people truly care, it is worth the effort."

Lieven: "I feel a bit like a preacher when I say this, but I want to end with an appeal: 'If it is so courageous for these people to start talking about it, we as their environment should be courageous enough to revisit the topic.' Ask a few weeks later how things are going and whether they still need to talk about it. This is like the situation with cancer patients. Everyone says, 'If you need me, just let me know.' The problem is that the sick person has to summon the courage to reach out. Wouldn't it be fairer for those who are not struggling so much to pick up the phone occasionally and ask? I notice the same with people who have lost a child. They tell me how hard it is to bring it up every time on their own. When someone asks after a year, 'Hey, how are you coping with Lizzy's loss?' that means everything. It's no different for those struggling with partner violence. Just share your courage with them."

Conclusion: silence is silver, speech is golden

In this chapter, we have aimed to convey some of the complexities involved in speaking about partner violence. The experience is layered and intertwined like an increasingly dense web. Each time, there is the story of one partner and the story of the other, the compelling dance of their interactions, and the couple's fragile inner world contrasted with the judgmental and concerned eyes of those around them—these are all forces that pull at the story and make speaking difficult. The next step often feels both within reach and yet further away. Shame thrives in this terrain. It is a slippery emotion that encourages hiding and withdrawal. When you hide, you may feel safe, but you are mostly alone. We hope that sincere encouragement reaches every reader. Each time courage triumphs over shame, there is a chance to truly see the person in front of you and for your partner to see you in return. Beyond shame lies the possibility that the couple's love can return to the light and become more openly expressed again.

Speaking up is a perilous undertaking, but it is undoubtedly worthwhile amid violence. And if it is difficult to find the courage for yourself, then do so for any (future) children growing up in the midst of that violence. It is about these children that we speak in the next chapter of this book, where we consider whether partner violence harms children.

Reflect and relate

Take a moment to pause and connect these ideas to your own experience.

Speaking about painful conflicts or moments of violence takes immense courage. These questions are not meant to push you but to gently help you notice what silence and speech mean in your own life—when you hide, when you speak, and what happens in between.

1. When you think about moments when things got out of hand, what makes it difficult for you to talk about them—with your partner, friends, family, or a therapist?

2. What fears hold you back from speaking—fear of judgment, rejection, losing love, or making things worse?

3. Are there people or places where you would feel safe enough to share even a small part of your story? What makes them feel safe?

4. How does shame show up for you when you try to talk about what happens between you and your partner?

5. What might change in your relationship if you could speak about your fears, pain, or shame without fear of being judged?

6
IS THIS HARMFUL TO OUR CHILDREN?

People who become entangled in escalating conflicts rarely feel good afterward. Once the peak of tension has subsided, a certain calm may return, but that's when the damage becomes visible. The broken dishes, the scratch on his arm, the bruise on her cheek, the hole in the door… and the emotional wounds that remain unseen. "Did I really say I'd rather live alone for the rest of my life than have sex with him one more time?" "I know she had a terrible childhood, and yet I told her she's even worse than her mother. How can I ever undo that?" "Calling him the least-involved father of the year was bad enough, but adding that my friends agree only made him feel more inadequate. Why did I have to put it so harshly?" When the realization of the damage hits, the pain is palpable, and then the guilt begins to gnaw.

For those who have children, or hope to have them someday, the question of harm—and the accompanying guilt—cuts even deeper. Children don't choose to be part of the conflict, yet they are inevitably affected by it. As parents, we often try hard to shield them from tension and escalation. "They were not in their room when things got loud, but they probably still heard us yelling." "He came to comfort me afterward, which was so sweet, but it's not right for my thirteen-year-old son to have to do that, is it?" "She took the blow that was meant for me. We both said it wasn't intentional, but will she ever

DOI: 10.4324/9781003683582-7

feel safe in our home again?" "After witnessing all this anger, how can they ever believe in love?" Any parent who loves their child, and who has experienced tension threatening to consume the household, will likely wrestle with questions like these. In this chapter, we focus on whether partner violence is harmful to children.

This chapter is somewhat of an outlier in its focus. Not all readers will have children. Some may not want them. Others may not yet feel ready. Still others may long for children but have been met with disappointment, knowing them only through the pain of unfulfilled desire. Many people enter relationships where children are already present—sometimes living with them, though not their biological parent—creating complex, often tense family dynamics. Similar challenges exist in families with foster children. We also consider parents of adult children who now find themselves witnessing their children's relationships spiral into conflict, worrying about the grandchildren growing up in such tension. And of course, many readers will have grown up in families marked by conflict and escalation. For all these reasons, it's worth writing about the effects of conflict on children—these vulnerable, yet remarkably resilient, human beings. At the same time, we recognize that this topic may be difficult or even painful for some readers. The choice is yours: skip ahead or read on.

Wise question; simple answer

The question of whether children are harmed by witnessing parental conflict troubles nearly all couples who struggle with intense arguments and who are also parents. For some, the question is a quiet undercurrent; for others, it's an anguished cry. But posing the question itself is wise. It reflects a growing awareness that the situation isn't ideal for the children. Asking means you care. It shows that you sense these escalations are not only affecting you and your partner—they are also affecting your children. In some families, children witness the conflict directly. In others, parents hope their children are shielded from it, but still wonder how much of the stress seeps through. There is often an implicit understanding that the tension is having an effect. The real question becomes: How much of an impact does it have, and is it lasting? Is there something we can do about it? In some heartbreaking instances, children intervene during acts of partner violence—sometimes even getting caught in the crossfire. In such cases, it's undeniable that they are harmed. Yet even then, parents are left wondering: Just how deep does the impact go, and what can we do to repair it? These reflections are full of care and concern.

Lieven: "In that respect, we can be quite clear: the answer is yes. Partner violence, and even more generally, ongoing household tension, has a negative impact on children. When a child sees or hears their parents argue, their body is filled with stress—and that takes a toll. Let me draw a parallel with divorce. Parents often ask how harmful divorce is for their children. But research shows that it's not the divorce itself that does the most harm—it's the fighting. The most harmful situation is when conflict continues before, during, and after the separation. In contrast, a divorce that ends the hostilities can actually be less damaging. It's the ongoing *tension that affects children most*. They are caught between two people who are both essential to them. When violence is added, it doubles the internal conflict and anxiety they experience."

Jef: "If you're worried about the impact of your escalations on your children, that's not only wise—it's also deeply caring. It shows that you're an engaged parent who wants what's best for your child. Our greatest hope is that both parents share this concern and can approach it TOGETHER. When that happens, the negative impact on children can sometimes be minimal. But when children are drawn *into* the conflict, the harm increases dramatically. This becomes a new kind of violence—parents, often unintentionally, using the child as a weapon in the struggle. For example: 'See how much you're hurting the kids by acting like this! What kind of parent are you?' Such tactics escalate the conflict and put the child in a deeply painful, confusing position. It tears at them."

Learning to play in the playground

Conflict between parents can be harmful to children. At the same time, children are remarkably resilient and often develop important skills in navigating such conflict. This creates a delicate balance. The metaphor of a playground is useful here: *the relationship between parents can be seen as the playground in which children grow up*. This romantic bond is typically characterized by a degree of emotional security, but it evolves over time and is shaped by numerous internal and external stressors. Children, both literally and figuratively, play within the emotional landscape of their parents' relationship. Within this space, they are exposed to examples, develop a range of skills, and accumulate countless formative experiences. When something is wrong in the parental relationship, children notice. The more conflict and strife there is, the less safe this playground becomes—and the higher the risk of emotional injury. At the same time, children often become remarkably adept at playing in their playground, even when it appears damaged or unstable to outsiders. This is a critical point. Partner violence is often described as a form of child abuse, and we do not dispute that it can impose a significant burden on children. Still, it is important to recognize that for many children, these situations are temporary. They also provide lessons on how to manage tension and conflict.

Jef: "There are children who grew up on playgrounds that were too safe—environments with no risk but also no challenge. In such settings, there's barely anything to play with. A ten-year-old, for example, isn't thrilled by a soft play area with only a half-meter-high slide and a rocking duck. If you grow up in a household where your parents never argued, it can be quite shocking the first time you have a dispute with someone you love. You haven't developed the calm or the skills to deal with that. So, a certain amount of risk is essential for learning how to play.

On the other hand, some children grow up in playgrounds that are permanently dangerous: rusty slides, loose bolts on the seesaw, cobblestones instead of soft ground, and a swing hanging by just one rope. It's astonishing how skilled children can become at playing in such environments. Their *resilience* is truly impressive. Don't ask me to swing from a single rope, but kids who grow up in that context can do it. Still, when the playground is chronically broken, children do get hurt. That's what happens to kids exposed to long-term, escalating conflict and violence. Yes, they develop certain skills, but growing up in such a setting is not a viable option. It leaves a heavy burden and causes lasting damage."

Lieven: "And then, of course, there are all kinds of playgrounds in between. That's where most children grow up—and where most partner relationships fall. These playgrounds offer a mix of safe and challenging equipment; sometimes something is broken and takes a while to fix, but there are also periods of joyful and secure play. In these spaces, children learn that conflict is a part of life—and that it can be resolved. When children see that there's tension at home, that their parents argue but then make up and restore peace, they learn how to *cope with emotional tension*. And because tension is part of life, this becomes a healthy component of their development."

Tension and conflict do affect children. But when these experiences are temporary and followed by recovery and reassurance, children acquire important coping skills. When conflict becomes chronic or escalates too frequently, those skills can be overshadowed by emotional harm. In such cases, resilience alone is not enough.

Through the eyes of the child

In earlier chapters, we described how couples build a house—and eventually a home—through many shared moments of "Finally!" Often, children are born into these homes, and it is where they grow up. In some families, the emotional atmosphere becomes charged with tension. When that tension ignites, the resulting explosion can shake the household to its foundation. We've already discussed what this means for the partners. But the children who live in that same house also experience the explosion—in their own way. To understand what parents can do in these situations, it's crucial to develop a deeper awareness of how children perceive conflict and escalation. What happens from the child's point of view when their parents lose control and lose each other during arguments?

Lieven: "It's not necessarily harmful for children to experience small earthquakes or explosions at home. These events can help them develop emotional coping strategies. They learn: 'The world can shake, there can be tension, and that will pass.' When these minor shocks occur, parents usually offer *comfort*: 'That was a bit intense, but it's over now. It's okay. Come here—you're not alone.' Through such reassurances, children learn to regulate their emotional responses. As long as they can still turn to their parents for comfort during moments of tension, they feel *protected*—even when the emotional ground trembles beneath them. Of course, it's not always easy for parents to offer comfort in the middle of a conflict, but often it's possible to do so afterward, once the most intense moment has passed: 'We argued, but it's okay now. We worked it out. That was a bit scary, wasn't it?'"

However, some explosions are much more intense. These include conflicts involving physical violence—pushing, pulling, objects being thrown—or emotionally charged shouting and blame. Long periods of cold, silent distance can feel just as seismic to a child. Regardless of the form, children feel the shockwaves and the tension. And more than adults, they need reassurance and protection. When children witness their protectors fighting in ways that shake the very structure of their home, the situation becomes deeply troubling. The place that should offer safety and protection suddenly becomes the source of danger. What are they supposed to do with that? This creates a *double insecurity*: the fear caused by the conflict itself, and the distress of not being able to turn to their parents for comfort. It's terrifying: our safe home is falling apart, and the people who are supposed to protect me are gone—or have become the danger themselves.

Children in the midst of parental conflict

Like adults, children facing overwhelming insecurity and fear have only two options: they move forward or retreat. A "step forward" can take many forms depending on the child's age—protesting, crying loudly, trying to distract their parents from each other, becoming involved in the conflict, or even physically placing themselves between fighting parents. A particularly striking form of this forward movement occurs when children begin to care for their parents: offering a listening ear, providing comfort, taking on practical responsibilities, or attempting to mediate. In doing so, they often suppress their own needs and boundaries, focusing instead on the emotional and practical needs of their distressed parents. In contrast, *stepping back* may look like hiding under the bed, standing silently on the stairs listening for the fight to end, retreating to their room, spending as much time as possible at a friend's house, or withdrawing quietly with a hood up and headphones on.

Lieven: "What that step forward or backward looks like depends on age. Being 2 years old or 18 makes a huge difference in how you experience violence between your parents. A two-year-old doesn't understand what's happening, but their body reacts with distress. They seek comfort from parents who are themselves upset—and that rarely works. This can become a dangerous combination. If you're in an escalating conflict and there are little ones crying and unable to soothe themselves, it doesn't exactly defuse the situation. Two-year-olds are also at the stage where they constantly test boundaries—saying 'No!' to everything. It wouldn't be surprising for them to react with that same resistance in response to the tension of a domestic conflict. This phase is challenging for any parent, let alone when you're feeling anxious, angry, and overwhelmed yourself.

By age 10, children already grasp quite a bit about what's going on during an escalating argument. Some will go out of their way not to make things worse—they may try extra hard at school, clean their rooms unprompted, or offer comforting words. Others may try to break the tension more directly: they might fight with a sibling, break things, yell, or act out at school or on the playground.

Adolescents respond differently. It's not uncommon for them to become actively involved in the conflict, stepping in to protect the more vulnerable parent. Some would rather absorb verbal or even physical blows themselves than watch one parent inflict harm on the other. Others may cope by withdrawing entirely—staying away from home as much as possible."

Regardless of age, these are all children who worry. Some do so more openly than others, as seen in the examples above. If a child expresses this worry out loud and you, as a parent, hear it, you have an important opportunity. Once the worst of the tension has passed and you feel calm and emotionally available again, return to it with your child. This might be hours later, a day later, a week, or even a month, but the sooner the better. Still, later is better than never. Revisit the moment. *Ask about it. Talk about it.* Children often voice their concerns in their own way. Think of the four-year-old who gently asks after a fight, "Are you friends again?" They are actively looking for reassurance. If possible, address this together with your partner: "We're worried. Things got out of hand, and that must have been hard for you, too. We weren't there for you—we were too caught up in our own anger and conflict. But now we're back, and we want to know how you're doing." It's perfectly normal to be unable to support your children in the heat of the moment. What matters is that your care and presence return. Make that care explicit. Name it, and invite your children to talk about what they experienced.

Vibrations without consolation

To help children manage the impact of partner violence, they need their parents. Parental care is essential. Once a parent can reengage in their parenting role, the experience of escalating conflict becomes far less overwhelming for the child. The parent's presence—as a parent—is a top priority for children. This makes it a shared challenge for communities and society to work with parents to help them resume their caregiving roles as soon as possible. In the context of partner violence, there is often a strong impulse to keep children away from their parents. Children naturally elicit our protective instincts. However, being separated from their parents only intensifies their greatest fear: "My parents are fighting, and now I've also lost my safe haven. My parents can't reassure me." Using the metaphor of a playground, our task is to *help parents restore the playground*. If they can make it safe again, children will naturally begin to play. But if we remove children from the playground altogether, we take away what was—and can be again—a safe place for them.

Jef: "This reminds me of Joy, a three-year-old boy and his six-year-old sister, Jarra. They live in a home filled with love, both for them and between their parents. Still, there are times when storms roll through their household. Their parents are a strong team, but they face heavy external pressures. They migrated to Belgium several years ago, and the weight of their family's expectations back in Malawi rests heavily on their shoulders. The health care of Joy and Jarra's grandfather depends on them. Financial stress, compounded by the loneliness of living in a cold, unfamiliar country, strains the warmth of their usual teamwork.

During these times, the father withdraws in silence, stepping outside, while the mother becomes angry, shouting about everything that's going wrong—all the failures. They fall into a familiar pattern described earlier in this book: one partner retreats further into emotional withdrawal, while the other escalates their attempts to reconnect, sometimes to the point of desperation. Eventually, the father, overwhelmed by a sense of failure, lashes out. He is a large, proud man; she is a small, delicate woman. Tension builds. He throws a bottle of water at the wall. Glass shatters. She screams louder: 'Do you feel like a man now? Do you think this is going to solve our problems?!' His hand flies and strikes her face. She falls to the floor, surrounded by shards of glass.

Joy stands in the doorway. He feels the earthquake tearing through his home. His small body absorbs the intensity of the violence. He trembles with fear. In this terrifying moment, he needs his parents. He wants to run to them, to be held and reassured. But he sees and hears the chaos coming from them, and he hesitates. He doesn't dare approach. His entire body is in a state of alarm. Naturally, he begins to cry."

At that point, many parents hear their child's crying and are jolted out of the cycle of violence. A child's distress can transcend conflict. The *parental instinct to protect reawakens*. That's what happens with Joy's father. He hears the crying, sees his little son frozen in fear, and immediately walks toward him. He picks Joy up and holds him. But something difficult occurs. Joy's small body is trembling, and his father's body is still vibrating with the after-shocks of rage and fear. Normally, the father can calm Joy by walking slowly, murmuring reassuring words. But this time, it doesn't work. Joy senses the lingering tension in his father's body. He sees his mother—now upright, but tending to her bleeding arm. There is no reassurance to be found. The trembling from his father only amplifies his own fear. He is also scared by the sight of blood. As his father's tension gets closer to him, it intensifies. Panic sets in: "My big, strong daddy, who always protects me, is different. He scares me."

Jef: "Joy begins to cry even harder. His father realizes he can't calm him and is flooded with self-reproach: 'Everything is going wrong. I love my wife so much, but I keep hurting her. She's sitting there in pain because of me. And now, I can't even comfort my son—my everything. He seems afraid of me. What kind of father am I?' You can feel how unsustainable this is. The tension is spiraling, and it's unbearable, especially for a child. So, something inside Joy shuts down. He turns off his 'vibrate button.' He stops reaching out. He withdraws entirely: 'I lock my fear inside my little body and shut myself off from the world.' This is a well-known protective strategy. Children learn it.

Meanwhile, Jarra enters the room. She takes her mother's hand and helps her up. 'Let's take care of you,' she says. On her way past Joy, she sees the fear in his eyes. She reassures him, 'It's not so bad. We'll put a plaster on it. It'll be fine. Go play.' She's only six, outwardly calm, but trembling inside. She copes with the stress in a very different way. She steps forward, taking charge, while turning off her own inner alarm. *'If I take care of everyone, eventually my parents will be able to help me deal with these strange and frightening feelings.'*"

Children who grow up using Jarra's strategy tend to take on responsibility during conflict. They step forward again and again—intervening, mediating, trying to restore peace. These actions are signals to their parents: "This isn't okay. Please stop fighting. Be gentle again." Children like Joy, on the other hand, learn a different response. "If I shut down and stay silent, the conflict eventually stops. Then my parents become available again. Until then, I just wait it out—alone." When Joy grows up and faces conflict in his own home, he might withdraw to his room. Or leave the house to visit friends. Above all, he won't ask questions or express his feelings. These children often seem unaffected, but they're not. They're locked inside a psychological bunker, filled with internal tension. They track the emotional climate with great sensitivity, listening from their rooms for the moment when the turbulence settles and it's safe to reconnect. They may appear absent, but they are profoundly alert.

Influence through care

One way children can exert some influence during conflict is through what might be called a "care-reflex." When a parent is absent, either physically or emotionally due to being caught in an argument, children often begin to care. This reflex provides them with a sense of agency amid chaos: even in the midst of losing control, they can do something. This caring can take many forms.

Lieven: "Becoming very well-behaved and sweet is one way of caring. There's already so much tension and burden in the house—I'm going to make sure it doesn't get worse. That links to children withdrawing or bunkering down. There's care in that. On the other hand, there's also active caring, like Jarra in the example Jef shared: comforting others, helping with household tasks, and keeping younger siblings occupied. In these moments, children step into a caregiving role, effectively reversing the parent–child dynamic. If the parent isn't providing care, then I will.

Sometimes, children even take responsibility for the relationship itself. They may try to mediate between their parents: 'Talk to each other. You can understand why she's acting that way. He still loves you, you know.' Concern for the relationship might also be expressed as: 'Just break up already. These fights are hurting you both. Stop it!' It's not uncommon for children to take sides. Usually, they support the more vulnerable parent. Sometimes, siblings divide their allegiances: You take Mom's side, I'll take Dad's. This is rarely discussed openly; it often happens implicitly. While it reflects deep care, it can come at a significant cost, especially when it results in sibling conflict. When that happens, children lose a vital source of mutual support.

Another form of care is seen in attention-seeking or disruptive behavior: 'If I destroy things, you'll have to deal with me—and

> maybe then you'll stop fighting.' In this way, children try to divert attention and assume the blame, motivated by concern for the family unit. All these behaviors—though divers—serve a common function: they allow children to exert some influence in the midst of emotional turmoil. Their caregiving gives them something to hold on to."

The underlying function of these various responses is to restore calm in the parents, in the hope that the parents will then be emotionally available and able to soothe the anxious, dysregulated child. Children *care in order to receive care.* Unfortunately, that care doesn't always follow. In this sense, their caregiving reflects a longing for comfort, security, and peace. It may be the only form of influence they have—and influence is vital. Influence fosters resilience. When a child feels they have some impact, it enhances their sense of security and agency.

Taking the burden and the concern seriously

Returning to the question, "Is this harmful to children?" the answer is both yes and no. It's akin to asking, "Is growing up harmful to children?" Growth, by its nature, involves some degree of pain. In this light, the word harmful may not be especially helpful. It carries an air of permanence and blame—as if something has been irreparably broken. This framing dishonors both the intentions of parents and the care they give, as well as the resilience that conflict often awakens in children. For this reason, we prefer terms like detriment or burden. Yes, witnessing intimate partner violence can certainly be detrimental to a child's development. At the same time, children can also develop skills as a result: coping with tension, building resilience, learning to tolerate conflict, and taking different perspectives. It may sound like a strange comparison, but people often say that experiencing cancer led them to grow as a person or as a couple. Of course, no one would suggest seeking out cancer. The same applies to frequent family conflict or violence: while children may grow from the tension, that doesn't mean we would ever recommend such circumstances.

Interestingly, parental guilt over what children experience can itself be a sign of something meaningful: care. It means the parent would rather have done things differently. We don't want to erase that guilt—because to do so would risk erasing the care it reflects. At the same time, we want to avoid blame, which similarly erodes the recognition of parental concern.

Lieven: "The question of whether violence harms children contains a lot of care. We want to encourage parents to *share that concern—with each other, and with their children*. If we've lost our way as parents, it's hard for children to find theirs, especially in moments of high stress. If we want to help the kids, the most important thing we can do is find each other again as parents—even if we can't do so as partners. 'Hey kids, that was loud, wasn't it? That was probably really stressful for you. Mom and Dad are going to try to work on that. It's okay that you were scared—for a moment, it *was* frightening.' Offering this kind of acknowledgment is the best form of care. It provides a path out of harm. Then the experience becomes a burden, but not one that must leave lasting scars. So let the care and concern in your question be expressed. Don't keep it to yourself. It can be deeply healing for children to hear this from their parents, especially when it comes from both of you together."

Helping parents to parent again

What happens when you, as part of the surrounding environment, are confronted with the suffering of children? When you suddenly gain insight into the lives of children inside a home that is shaking at its foundations, it may be the first time you truly see the insecurity they live with or sense a little of the emotional storm they are caught in. That realization can be jarring. Naturally, you feel a strong urge to protect the children. You want to remove them from this danger, to lift the burden from their shoulders. But what we often forget is that, before a house begins to shake visibly, many smaller tremors have already occurred within it. For the children, this may not be a new experience. Is this stressful for them? Of course. Everyone agrees on that: the children, the surrounding environment, and the parents. The problem is that the parents are often so deeply entangled in the conflict that it becomes difficult for them to function as parents. When outsiders notice this, they often emphasize how damaging the situation is for the children. But most parents already know this. Repeating it only adds to their sense of failure, reducing the mental space they have to actually parent.

Jef: "When it comes to the impact on children, it's important to remember that while the 'earthquake' of violence frightens them, what truly terrifies them is losing their source of comfort and security. If we want to protect children, we need to *prioritize their greatest* *fear*: the loss of their parental base is more overwhelming than the conflict itself. It is crucial that children regain their source of safety and reassurance as quickly as possible. That source is, ideally, their parent—at least to the extent that is feasible. 'I often refer to Patricia Crittenden, an American psychologist who did a lot of research around attachment and developmental psychology.' She says, 'Treat parents the same way you would want them to treat their children.' If parents are overwhelmed by the conflict and the emotional turmoil it creates, we—as the surrounding environment—can show them that we recognize they don't want things to be this way. We can offer them a space where they can find warmth, catch their breath, and begin to calm down. This helps them become regulated again—meaning their own emotions no longer dominate them, and they can once again take the wheel. Only then can they begin to do the same for their children."

Lieven: "The environment can also play a temporary but important role for the children. We can be a *source of comfort* and stability until the parents are able to resume that role. But this only works if the children sense that their parents are not being condemned or dismissed. Otherwise, their greatest fear resurfaces: 'I've lost my main source of comfort and protection.' "Children are deeply loyal. They can only accept support from others if there is still space for their parents in the narrative. We might say something like, 'It's hard when your mom and dad fight like that, isn't it? That probably made you really scared. That's okay. We're going to give them a little time to make up. They don't want it to be this way either. In the meantime, I'm here with you.'"

The goal is clear: if we want to reduce children's exposure to parental conflict or violence, we must help parents resume their role as reassuring and protective caregivers as quickly as possible. This is about being present again as a parent—even if they have not reconciled as partners. These are two distinct processes, each moving at its own pace. A parent might say, "We can't resolve this between us right now, but we can try to stay present for the children—or do something to make sure we can be there for them as parents. And if we couldn't be there, we'll try to repair that with the children afterward." In these situations, the principle of *better late than never* applies. Many adults, even at age 35, are deeply moved when a parent finally says, "It must have been really hard for you and your brother when we fought so much." Even though the child has long since left the conflict behind, being acknowledged still carries enormous healing power. Never underestimate the impact of recognition: "We weren't there—not because you weren't worth it, but because we were too caught up in our own conflict."

The inner world of the parent

Previously, we reflected on what happens to children when they become involved in parental conflict. But what about the parents? What happens to them—and within them—when the children become part of the conflict? The dynamics of partner violence are complex, but they become even more intricate when the partners are also parents. Across the previous pages, it has become clear that such violence often stems from two primary disruptions: the loss of security in the relationship, which may lead to distance-seeking aggression, and the loss of connection, which can trigger proximity-seeking aggression. Together, these forces can cause emotional earthquakes—storms that shake a home and leave it cracked and torn. In the midst of one of these storms, you might stomp out of a room and head upstairs—only to suddenly encounter your two children sitting on the steps. Their shoulders are raised, their eyes wide with fear. The older child holds her hands over her younger sibling's ears, trying to shield him from the noise. They are just as startled by the encounter as you are. No matter what role you occupy in the couple's pattern of conflict, this moment shakes your identity as a parent.

One person might feel, "I can't even manage as a partner—now I'm failing as a parent too." Another might think, "I already felt so alone. I can't turn to my partner… and now I see that my children are afraid of me—because of me. I'm ruining everything. I'll be alone forever." Whatever attachment wounds you carry, the look in your *children's eyes cuts straight through you.* It deepens the pain already caused by the conflict and pushes your sense of powerlessness to new heights. In that moment, the capacity to provide parental care is still there, but it is buried under layers of distress and emotional overload.

Jef: "When your ability to parent is blocked like that, we often see it resurface in a distorted form. You might shout, 'Look what you're doing! It's not enough that I'm falling apart—now you're destroying the children too!' Here, *parental concern becomes a weapon in the conflict.* Instead of letting your care speak for itself, you point out the damage from a defensive stance.

In the family I mentioned earlier, it might sound like, 'Look, now you've made Joy cry too!' The shared care that could help us respond differently as parents is swallowed up by powerlessness and becomes more fuel for the conflict. If you have a mother's or father's heart, and your partner accuses you of being a bad parent, it's unbearable. It's no surprise that such accusations can escalate the cycle of violence.

I think this illustrates how overwhelming these emotions are. In such moments, we cannot expect to function constructively, either as partners or as parents. That comes later, after the storm."

Lieven: "There's another dynamic at play—another way we lose ourselves and each other in the storm or the quake. You see the children's eyes, and it breaks your parental heart because this is exactly what you never wanted your child to experience. In response to that pain, you may lash out and blame the other parent. But remember, inside every adult parent, there is also a child. And sometimes, that child experienced similar trauma growing up. In the eyes of their children on the stairs, parents may suddenly see a reflection of themselves: sitting in fear, taking the blows, comforting a parent after a violent episode… and vowing that their own children would never have to go through that. And yet, here they are. That buried childhood experience adds a second layer to the emotional burden, making it nearly impossible to remain in a parental role. The storm has to pass first. The emotional tremors must subside. Only then can the parent re-emerge—present, attuned, and responsive."

What Jef and Lieven describe makes it easy to understand why parents don't calmly turn to each other and say, "Hey, what are we doing? This isn't good for the kids. How can we change this?" Instead, what happens is loud, defensive, accusatory. In the chaos, you hear the children's crying—or suddenly catch a glimpse of a tear-streaked face or terrified eyes. Seeing that child's body awakens the memory of your own child-body. You think, *This is the last thing I ever wanted. How did I get here?* Inside, you may feel an urge to say, "We have to stop. This isn't good for the children." But fear takes over, and instead, you turn to your partner and say, "This got so out of control because you don't communicate and keep ignoring me!" Or, "It's because you're always criticizing and giving me no space!" More fuel. More fire. More conflict.

The time of/for recovery

This summary of suffering makes it clear that it is impossible to provide proper care as a parent during a violent escalation. You know you want to care, but you simply cannot reach that place. We want to offer everyone here the gift of *time*. It may not work during the escalation, but after time has done its work, you will be able to care. Don't let that opportunity pass. Because then your children will need you, and you can stand together as parents.

A storm does not last forever. It always subsides—eventually—even if only temporarily. The period after the storm is a time when recovery is possible.

Jef: "Your own body trembles for a while and then gradually settles more completely. Often, adults in this phase are so busy tending to their own wounds that they forget the children's bodies are still trembling just as much. Children need you very much in that moment. Focus on your children then. Even if you thought they were asleep during the conflict but noticed their deep silence at breakfast. Even if they were at school when you clashed, the bruise hadn't healed by the time they started their homework and couldn't concentrate. Comfort them and reassure them until their trembling fades."

Lieven: "Many parents think, after a violent outburst, 'Now everything has to be fun, safe, and cozy! The tension must disappear. No more talking about it. We'll put it in a big box and store it away.' It's understandable to want only to think about pleasant things once the earthquake is over. It's also understandable not to want to talk about the conflict again for fear it will flare up. Still, we strongly encourage you to revisit the issue with your children: 'That was intense, wasn't it? How are you feeling now? Do you still need comfort?'"

If you are wondering whether incidents of violence harm children, take your concern seriously. Seize the opportunity to address it when it is possible—that is, after the storm. You cannot undo the storm, but you can undo the fact that you disappeared as a parent. You can re-emerge as a caregiver by explicitly acknowledging that the child's body—big or small—is still trembling: "I see you're shaking. Come here. Tell me." Many people believe that talking about painful things will reopen wounds. In reality, it is being alone with that pain that weighs most heavily on people, especially children. So engage in the conversation, even if it takes a great deal of courage from parents. Children are worth that courage.

What do you want to teach children about tension?

Why is it so important to find the courage and make time afterward to talk with children about what happened? Returning to the trembling in the body when things are calm matters not only in the here and now. In the immediate moment, it helps children find peace and rest. Over the long term, it has an impact throughout their development. If parents decide, "We're not going to talk about it anymore because now it's calm and we don't want to wake the storm," the vibration remains in the body, and children must manage it on their own. As you know, they have only two options: to bunker down in pain or to protest and scream out in pain elsewhere.

Jef: "Children in the first group tend to develop an avoidant strategy for dealing with tension. Those in the second group adopt a more clinging strategy. The 'bunkerers' learn, *'I can't count on others; I have to reassure myself.'* They struggle with even minor tension and differences in many types of relationships. They also store small vibrations in their bunker. These stored vibrations can show up in very different ways: difficult behavior at school, learning difficulties, feelings of depression, trouble concentrating, and so on. As these children grow, they continue signaling, 'Help! I still need parental care to calm these stored vibrations.' However, the way they express this often becomes hard to understand. As they mature, there is a risk they become trapped in this avoidant or withdrawn position. They often become highly sensitive to tension but have difficulty expressing what they truly need."

Lieven: "The second group, the protesting children, feel, *'The other isn't there for me, so I'll do whatever it takes to be heard and to reach the other person.'* These children are often described as seeking negative attention. Their stored vibrations tend to manifest as outbursts of anger, loud and hyperactive behavior, or clinginess—they constantly seek attention and struggle to be alone. Yet they, too, are still seeking comfort and reassurance. Again, it is often difficult to recognize that these symptoms reflect very different underlying stress. As these children mature, we frequently find them in a pursuing position. They remain very sensitive to rejection and seek confirmation in various ways that the other person is present and will stay with them."

For now, we describe these patterns in two broad terms, but of course, this is not a black-and-white story—there are many shades of gray. We are describing a general direction and effect, and for clarity's sake, have left out many other influences in growing up: peers, family, life events, and hobbies. These elements also affect tension, vibrations, and the development of withdrawing or pursuing strategies. The bottom line is this: if we don't return to the issue, we teach children that returning is not possible. Then they are left alone with their tension, which will eventually find another way out.

Jef: "Inside all adults caught in violent interactions live trembling children. As adults, they promise themselves, 'That will never happen to my children. They will never see me furious. They will grow up in a home without violence.' And yet, there comes a moment when they say, 'Damn! That's the last thing I wanted for my children, and now it's happening anyway… I'm creating a storm for my children too. If we still carry many unresolved vibrations from our own childhood, it is an illusion to think we can fully protect our children from them. After all, children live very close to us. They feel that storm inside. They collide with it. The promise that your children will never experience this is too great a promise. Perhaps we can work toward a situation where, if your children do encounter your storm, *you can be there for them afterward so that they are left with fewer vibrations—and so their own children in turn won't have to go through this*. You can make that difference. That is part of 'good enough parenting.' It is a realistic expectation. When escalating conflicts occur, if you take the time afterward to calm your child's body, they won't grow up to be adults burdened by bunkered or constantly vibrating tension."

Conclusion: yes, it is detrimental and yes, you can do something about it

Parents who argue cannot shield their (potential) children from the accompanying tension—no matter how much they want to. Because children and parents share the same house, they experience this tension together. While children do learn valuable skills for managing tension by witnessing conflict, frequent or prolonged exposure to such tension takes a toll on them. In those moments, they need their parents to help lift that burden from their shoulders. Unfortunately, during conflicts, parents are often too overwhelmed to provide that reassuring and protective presence.

The fact that you ask yourself, "Is this harmful to our children?" shows that you are an engaged parent who cares deeply about your children. This question creates an opportunity for change. Although this situation was the last thing you wanted for your children, it has become their reality. History seems to be repeating itself, and you may feel powerless. However, by asking the question, you have already reclaimed some influence: you see it, you feel it, you understand it. Imagine if your parents—despite their disagreements—had regularly taken the time to sit down with you and say, "How is this affecting you? We never wanted you to go through this, but it happened, and it scares you. Maybe it makes you angry. We don't have all the answers yet, but we will keep working together so that this no longer weighs on you. What do you need to feel reassured?" That is where the cycle is broken, allowing children's bodies to relax again and easing the impact on their development and on any future children.

No matter how overwhelming conflict is for adults and children, parents can ultimately let their love win the battle in which their children are unintentionally caught. This support helps children in the present and nurtures their growth into adults who will fight for love more safely.

Speaking of children brings us to the future. Couples who often find themselves stuck in conflict naturally have many questions about the future of their relationship. Will this continue? Will we ever get out of it? Can the future hold something different for me and for us? We address these concerns in the seventh and final question.

Reflect and relate

Take a moment to pause and connect these ideas to your own experience.

Parenting in the midst of conflict can be deeply painful. These questions are not about blame, but about awareness—noticing what your children might experience, and what you long to offer them.

1. When conflict arises at home, what do you think your children see, hear, or feel in those moments? How do you imagine their bodies respond when voices rise or silence stretches too long?

2. Can you recall a time when your child sought closeness after a fight—perhaps by comforting you or asking if everything was "okay"? What did that moment awaken in you?

3. When tension fades, what helps you return to your parental role—to reengage as a source of calm and care?

4. Are there moments when you sense that your own childhood experiences echo in how you now respond to your children's fear or distress?

5. How do you and your partner (or co-parent) usually talk to your children after conflict? What might they need to hear from you?

   If you could tell your child one thing after a painful argument, what would it be? If you picture yourself doing this, how does it make you feel as a parent?

7
WILL THIS FIGHT EVER END?

As we near the end of this book, it is natural that questions about the conclusion of escalations arise. When one frequently finds themselves caught in a dynamic that begins with love and good intentions but can deteriorate into something as destructive as violence, it is unsurprising that despair sometimes takes hold. Repeatedly cycling through violence feels like a rollercoaster of fast-paced interactions and intense emotions—essentially, a war of attrition. Understandably, people then ask themselves, "Will this fight ever end?"

This question can be heard in many ways, as it contains multiple underlying concerns: Will the violence stop? Will it stop on its own? If not, what can be done? Can we, as a couple, find a way to reverse this dynamic, or is that unrealistic in a relationship where violence (at times) occurs? Would it be better for me to leave and move on alone? But if I leave, am I bringing this dynamic with me, potentially repeating it in the next relationship? Or isn't it preferable for both of us to find a way out of this destructive labyrinth? Like many complex issues, one question begets another, creating a seemingly endless cycle.

The mental turmoil of people facing partner violence often feels grinding and exhausting. One thing is clear: partners do care deeply about what is happening. They tirelessly search for ways to end the violence. However, their

DOI: 10.4324/9781003683582-8

efforts do not always produce the peace they seek. In the following chapter, we explore the many layers and questions embedded in the query, "Will this ever stop?"

The spontaneous stop

Two important words stand out in this chapter's question: *ever* and *stop*. The word *ever* reflects the profound powerlessness people feel when trapped in patterns of violence. The word *stop* reveals what they truly want—they do not want violence in their relationship. Regardless of their role in the conflicts, no one desires violence. Yet, apparently, it persists. The fact that you are reading this book indicates you want to understand what is happening and are willing to do something different—that you are saying, "I don't want this!"

Like many previous questions, this one expresses a desire: a wish to gain better control over escalations and to find ways to prevent situations from spiraling out of control. There is no simple yes-or-no answer. People want to have, or at least feel, some influence over violent escalations. We hope this book will help foster that sense of control.

The first aspect we address is the natural or spontaneous end of violence. In fact, many couples experience violence that ends on its own. Simply wanting more peace and control over conflicts can spark a drive to change, often leading to the automatic cessation of violence.

Lieven: "The people discussed in this book are those struggling with situational partner violence. The readers themselves do not accept what is happening and are figuring out how to stop it. Sometimes people manage this on their own. They often find a way to act differently spontaneously because they are *shocked by how they see themselves, their partner, and their relationship* at the moment conflict escalates to violence. They think, 'Oh my! Is this what I'm doing? What does that say about who I am? What is my partner doing right now? Is this who we are as a couple? Is this the relationship we want?' People are startled by the clear escalation and the image they see of themselves and the other person. The brakes come on: 'We don't want this anymore!' Often, that alone is enough to prompt meaningful change."

A common belief in society is: "Once violence occurs in a relationship, it always continues and only worsens." However, the scientific literature does not support this view. Many people wake up after the first incident, thinking, "This is a red line we crossed, and it will never happen again!" For example, American researchers (Feld & Strauss, 1989) have shown that in 33%–58% (Aldarondo, 1996) of couples who experience violence, it stops spontaneously. Another study (Jasinski, 2001) followed couples over five years and found that violence ceased spontaneously in 70% of these relationships. It is important to distinguish three groups within this 70%: couples where violence stops but relational dynamics remain unchanged; couples where violence ends because they separate; and couples where violence stops because they successfully address and improve underlying dynamics. A relevant quote from similar research (Merchant & Whiting, 2017) states: "For most couples, ending violence was only part of their story. They didn't necessarily want to end the violence, but to change their whole lives: improve their relationship, become better individuals and find stability. All of these changes resulted in stopping the violence."

Jef: "You often see spontaneous disengagement in what I call 'tic-tac-toe couples.' Maybe you know a pair like this in your circle of friends or family. These are couples who are constantly bickering. Within 10 minutes of meeting them, they're at it:

> *'We went to the beach on Friday-'*
> *'No! That was Saturday.'*
> *'I'm telling you it was Friday. I'd just taken the car to the carwash.'*
> *'That was Saturday! You've got a hole in your head, you.'*
> *'Oh, listen to her! As if I don't remember when I wash my own car.'*

And so it goes. As an outsider, it can be hard to understand how they tolerate each other. Yet Gottman—an American psychologist and researcher who does a lot of research on couples and what (doesn't) work in a relationship—describes beautifully how these couples not only argue frequently but also make up and express affection just as often. They're couples marked by strong differences and high emotional intensity. What matters is the ratio of negative to positive interactions. As irritating as their dynamic may seem to others, if that ratio is balanced, the frequent bickering can actually work. When you ask these couples about a specific argument, and they immediately start debating what day it happened, you know: one partner lost the connection on Friday, the other on Saturday. What they want is to be understood. The emotional

> tension builds in that struggle. One partner insists it was Friday, and the other feels invalidated, pushing even harder to assert their version of events. Eventually, the tension becomes so overwhelming that they can no longer articulate it in words. Instead, they try to express their experience physically. In this context, physical expression, whether a raised voice or even a slap, signals that something needs attention. It jolts them into awareness: 'Oh no, this is going too far. Time out. We need to pause, take a breath, and start over. Time to be kind again.'

For these couples, the *violence can be understood* as a form of feedback. In therapy, they often say, 'Sometimes we push things to the limit or even cross it, but then we stop. When we're face to face, we know we have to pull back. We do that together.' In this context, the violence becomes a signal—an indication that helps them shift toward something more constructive. When both partners recognize that things are going too far, there's often a shared look that conveys, "We don't want this, do we?" and the response, "No, we don't." Together, they stop—because of *and* through the violence. That sense of togetherness is essential.

The road together or the road alone

In addition to couples who escalate symmetrically—where crossing the line into violence becomes a wake-up call that helps them stop—there are also couples in which things get so out of hand that one partner becomes deeply afraid. In these cases, aggression is not interpreted as a mutual signal to halt; instead, it is seen as "too dangerous." The implicit message becomes: "Our train of arguments… it could take us to a very ugly destination, so we must avoid it at all costs from now on." These individuals lose the courage to take the emotional risk of engaging in disagreement or expressing difference. They *no longer trust themselves or their partner to de-escalate* in time. The question "Is it ever going to stop?" becomes ingrained in the dynamics of the relationship, as one partner is no longer confident that conflict will remain within safe boundaries. As a result, they adopt an avoidant position. As we explained earlier, this dynamic can trap the couple in a new—pattern—one in which one partner pursues, while the other withdraws. Unfortunately, this pattern still holds the potential for violence. While one partner avoids conflict in an effort to preserve safety, the other becomes increasingly anxious and begins to demand more connection and clarity.

The pursuing partner feels the growing distance and sense of loss, which intensifies their fear and leads them to knock harder on the emotional door. These are the couples who rarely manage to escape this level of escalation on their own. They often need external help to learn how to argue in a different, less violent way.

When violence becomes a wake-up call, two paths emerge: the road together or the road alone. We want to encourage all readers of this book to consider taking the road together. If you care about each other but fear that your conflicts may spiral into violence, the road together requires a willingness to look inward and, possibly with outside support, gain a *shared understanding of what is happening between you*. How do we get from that sense of "Finally!"—that rush of being heard or released—to the pain we end up inflicting on each other, and ourselves? From that awareness, you can begin to search for emotional safety, which must accompany the path toward physical safety. Finding a skilled couples therapist can be a valuable resource in this process. Still, it must be a mutual effort, and it starts with confronting your own boundary: "We don't want this," followed by a shared commitment to work on it together.

Some, however, choose the road alone at this point: "If we keep hurting each other like this, maybe we're simply not meant to be. We can't make it safe for one another, so it's better to part ways."

Lieven: "The road alone comes with important caveats. Sometimes, it is not a genuine decision but rather part of the same destructive interaction cycle. It can be an expression of despair or even a threat: 'If you keep nagging me like this, I'm done! I can't live with you anymore!' When said to a partner who fears abandonment, this only fuels anxiety and escalates the conflict. In such cases, the statement is part of the dangerous dance in which the couple is trapped. That is different from truly choosing the road alone.

The genuine road alone is a conscious decision to end the relationship from a place of calm. We sometimes see this in couples therapy. Some couples journey together in therapy, learn to be more safely connected, and reach a place of emotional calm. *In that calm, they may come to a mutual realization*: 'We understand each other well enough now to know that we will always trigger violence in each other. We don't want that, so it's better to go our separate ways.' Do you see how this can be a safe—and even connected—way to end a relationship?"

The silence *after* the storm

There are many ways to stop violence. At the same time, every couple that struggles with violent conflict is, in some way, constantly stopping it. After a violent episode, any couple not experiencing intimate terrorism will feel, "We don't want that anymore." After something gets broken, both partners may be shocked and begin trying to explain things more calmly. A blow is struck and one of them walks away. After a bout of pushing and pulling that ends in a fall, concern over the injury brings the escalation to a halt. For some couples, this takes longer than for others, but eventually there is always a pause—a silence, a moment of calm. A stopping always follows. In extreme cases, this happens because one person simply stops moving. So there is a continual, though temporary, stopping. Yet tension inevitably begins to build again, setting the stage for potential new violence. In this phase, both partners may wonder, "Are we going to keep slipping on this same icy surface?" That wondering, too, is a kind of pause.

Jef: "The paradox is that we keep slipping on the same ice because we keep falling into the same interaction patterns—relying on the same protective strategies and reaching the same point where we try to stop. Imagine the man who, after an escalation that leaves bruises, says to himself, 'I'm never stepping on that ice again!' and begins avoiding all conflict. Meanwhile, his partner may be thinking, 'We desperately need to learn how to skate on this ice. If we keep falling, we need to practice until we can stay upright.' We've talked before about the attachment needs that lie beneath these behaviors. But there's another layer of meaning here: everyone is searching for their own way to avoid getting hurt again. *Each person has a personal strategy to stop the cycle of violence.* But the harder they try to stop it on their own, the more entangled they become. These are couples who are not trying to stop it *together*. Each is fighting for their own solution. They're making enormous efforts, but what they need is something different to stop the violence permanently."

When we reflect on the kinds of behaviors or habits people can stop fairly easily, they tend to be those that are not too emotionally charged—or those we understand well. Quitting snacks and stopping nail-biting—these are achievable when there's not a strong emotional undercurrent. But when intense emotions are involved, stopping requires a deeper understanding of what's happening both internally and relationally. What triggers it? What does it evoke in me? What is my typical reaction? What forces are at play? What impact does it have? These questions are just as relevant when it comes to patterns of violence. Only by gaining insight into yourself in relation to the other person can you begin to influence and change these patterns.

Lieven: "Think about people who slap their partner, feel ashamed afterward, and promise themselves it will never happen again. If they don't understand what triggers them so strongly, what role they play in the cycle, and how they and their partner fuel each other's responses—then no matter how sincere their intentions, they won't gain control over those slaps. If you don't feel your way through this process, you risk being overwhelmed again. There's a real danger that the same thing will happen because you didn't see it coming. Your emotions will be faster than your awareness, so you need to become intimately familiar with them. Without that, the violence can overtake you again. *Stopping means understanding yourself, understanding the other, and understanding the event between the two of you.* It also means learning to be compassionate toward yourself: 'When that happens, I get so scared and feel so much pain. I feel powerless and speechless. And then something overwhelms me that makes me do things I don't want to do. I say things that I know will hurt my partner deeply. My hand lashes out. I push him…'"

Recognizing the pattern

People want the violence to stop. Only a very small percentage are unwilling to let go of it—and those people are not reading this book. For many, the violence ends on its own, simply because they cross a certain threshold. But for many others, it doesn't stop, despite their best efforts. For them, togetherness becomes crucial. The question becomes: How can we walk this path together so that the cycle of violence is broken and escalations remain ordinary quarrels? When we walk that path together, we begin to understand that partner violence speaks more about the dynamics between us than about individual actions alone. Whether we both engage in physical aggression or one of us inflicts harm through words or silence, the buildup happens between us. We're engaged in a shared struggle—to manage the tension, to protect ourselves from pain, to preserve a sense of safety, to try to save the relationship.

But we fight separately, and we both end up hurt. When we begin to understand, both in ourselves and in each other, what drives us to fight, what we are fighting for, and how we are fighting, then space opens up for something new. Sometimes, things escalate so quickly that even if you want to stop, you can't. But as you become more attuned to yourself, to your partner, and to the relationship dynamic, the pace begins to slow. You start to notice what's happening, as it's happening. And together, you begin to recognize, "We're doing it again, aren't we?" That moment offers a real chance—as a couple—to break the spiral.

Jef: "Let's make this concrete with a couple's story: Frank and Isabella. Frank shared with me: 'We've been sleeping apart for a month now—ever since the incident. Things have been calm since then, and we're doing well with the children. But I still find it difficult that we're not sleeping in the same bed. We haven't had a conflict in weeks, but every night, the whole scene replays in my mind. The reason I'm lying there alone, the blood on her cheek, the fear in her eyes… I feel so guilty. I completely lost control and really hurt her. Since then, Isabella has been afraid of me, and she won't be in the room where it happened. I never want to hurt her like that again.' Frank is deeply preoccupied with the incident and its impact. He is determined not to let it happen again: 'I truly don't want that ever again. And yet, last week, it almost happened. I nearly broke my teeth trying not to explode. It took everything I had, but I managed to hold it in.' When I asked what helped him keep control, Frank said, 'It was actually Isabella who helped me stop.'"

Isabella's previous partner left her for another woman after several affairs. She knows what it feels like to be abandoned. She also never knew her father, and when her mother died five years ago, the fear of being alone began to overwhelm her regularly. Whenever Frank is late—coming home from work, from the bakery, or from visiting his mother—her anxiety flares up. She becomes highly reproachful. For Frank, it was always hard to understand the intensity of her accusations. When they became too long, too intense, or too frequent, his withdrawn silence would eventually give way to explosive *anger fueled by a desperate need for space*.

Jef: "No matter how strongly Frank resolves not to be aggressive again, the relationship dynamic often pushes him toward that edge. Just a few days ago, Isabella's fear of abandonment resurfaced. Once again, the accusations returned: 'You don't care about me at all! You only care about yourself!' As the reproaches continued, Frank felt increasingly trapped. He finally shouted, 'I don't want this! You know I don't want this! Stop!' In that moment, Isabella remembered our therapy sessions, where we had explored how Frank's 'Stop!' doesn't mean he wants to leave her—it means he doesn't want to hurt her. It reflects his desire to do right by her, to preserve the relationship, and his deep concern for how she sees him. She felt the echo of those moments when he had been able to explain this calmly. And yet, the fear still surged through her. So she asked, sharply, 'Do you want to get away from me, or do you want to stop this from going wrong again?' At that, Frank felt a wave of tension release: 'Of course I want to be with you. I just want peace. I want this ugly, painful conflict to end. I don't want to become that monster from last time.' Isabella fell silent. She went outside to the garden and lit a cigarette. In the quiet that followed, Frank's breathing slowed. With each breath, the threat of the aggression he had been battling inside began to fade further into the background."

The story of this couple shows us how two people can move from being overwhelmed individually to reaching a new kind of together. This isn't a romantic ideal of unity, but rather a shared understanding—of themselves, each other, and the relational patterns that hijack them. Sometimes, it only takes one partner in the moment to remember this and make it visible. That awareness becomes a doorway back to connection. It's a reciprocal process: knowing yourself and regulating your own emotions, while also knowing the other and learning how to co-regulate together.

Putting the whole puzzle together

The dynamics that emerge when we become afraid of losing love or security are often rooted in painful experiences from earlier in life. In these moments, the need for protection can feel urgent and overwhelming. Paradoxically, however, any form of self-protection often fuels escalation, thereby increasing the risk of violence. When individuals begin to recognize and understand this interplay, they shift from feeling powerless to feeling more empowered. They are no longer ambushed or hijacked by their emotional responses, and this awareness helps to calm the fearful brain.

Lieven: "In addition, it helps to make space to understand the violence—however damaging it was—and to listen to what that aggression was trying to communicate. This creates room to face the burden, the cost, and the harm, and to be able to say, as Frank did, 'I hurt you deeply. I didn't mean to. But I did. And now, of course, you're scared.' That's when both people begin to *see, feel, and acknowledge the damage, while simultaneously connecting with the relational function of the aggression*, whether it was an attempt to seek closeness or to create distance. Both parts are necessary. If either the harm or the underlying function is denied, the protest will inevitably return. But when both are acknowledged, more space and peace can emerge. We see in practice that when couples begin to recognize this and talk about it, they develop the capacity to deal with their sense of powerlessness. In such cases, the compulsion toward violence diminishes."

When couples find language for the attachment-related distress underlying their conflicts, they begin to express those needs more directly: "I need your closeness. I need your safety. I need you to see how hard I work for you. I need you to see how important your presence and care are to me." *Talking about these emotions prevents the silence in which physical expressions often take over.*

Jef: "We hope this book helps you discover that language together. We're also convinced that relationship counseling—contrary to popular belief—is the best way to find that shared path. It's much more difficult to build a shared story when therapy is done separately or individually.

Think of the many anger management or emotion regulation programs. These can be incredibly helpful because they address a crucial piece of the puzzle. But a single puzzle piece doesn't complete the picture. When you do this work as a couple, you not only gain insight into your own internal world but also into your partner's, and into how those worlds interact—often triggering a cycle of violence. And then you begin to see all the smaller pieces connected to that interaction. So our advice is to seek counseling that focuses on connection: connection to your own pain and connection between you as partners."

Quitting, relapsing, and quitting

There is clearly a path toward greater understanding and less escalation and violence. At the same time, relapse is possible. It's similar to what happens with alcohol addiction: people may stop drinking for a week, two weeks, several months, even years—and then relapse.

This is due to a kind of neurological vulnerability. Once the brain has discovered a quick path to reduce stress, that pathway remains accessible. The same is true for violence. Once a person has developed the neural association between powerlessness, wordlessness, and violent response, that connection exists. Under intense external stress or when verbal communication breaks down, a relapse may occur. A resurgence of violence is always jarring, but it does not mean that all previous efforts were futile.

Lieven: "*The question is whether relapse marks the end of the relationship*. For some, it does. They may say, 'We'll never fully get this under control. I can't go on. This was one time too many. We need to break up.' And indeed, working toward a future without violence is worthwhile. For some, the relapse is a turning point and signals the end of the relationship. It may be a wise and responsible decision to conclude together, 'We're too dangerous a combination. Let's take care of ourselves—and each other—by ending the relationship.' In that case, each person moves forward alone. For others, the fact that the violence had been absent for a long time may reassure them that it can be brought under control again. They might say, 'We know the way to peace and safety; we'll find it again, and faster this time.' These couples re-examine what triggered the relapse—perhaps unresolved pain or intense external pressures—and, in doing so, they gain a deeper understanding of the overall dynamic. Both responses are valid."

Some couples caught in entrenched relational patterns—or, at the extreme, in violent relational patterns—choose to separate, and in doing so, stop the violence. This is a completely valid path. However, one important caveat deserves attention: just as a divorce prompted by persistent conflict can devolve into a legal battle (and thus perpetuate the conflict), ending a relationship marked by partner violence does not always end the violence. In cases such as stalking, for instance, the underlying emotional wounds and attachment needs, whether for contact or distance, may be further activated when one partner decides to separate. Additionally, when children are involved, the partners must continue to interact in some capacity, and those ongoing interactions can reactivate familiar patterns of violence.

The road alone

Even when walking the road alone, it remains profoundly meaningful to understand and attune to three essential "puzzle pieces": *what is happening inside of me, what is happening inside the other person, and how these two inner experiences connect in a predictable, recurring dance between us*. Once both partners come to know and share these patterns, choosing to walk the road alone can emerge from a place of mutual understanding and peace. It becomes a kind of shared decision: We understand what we do to each other, and we know that we will continue to do so… so being apart is the best we can do.

"If I am truly myself, I will always be too loud and too much for you. If I am truly myself, I will always be too quiet and too little for you. We now recognize that this difference will always be a source of tension. There is nothing inherently wrong with this difference. At the beginning, we didn't even notice it—or it may have even drawn us together. But we are fundamentally built too differently." Reaching this point of awareness can bring emotional relief and a sense of freedom in choosing the road alone. It becomes clear that a kind of togetherness in separation is both possible and, in some cases, preferable. At the same time, we must acknowledge that this is not always easy or achievable.

Jef: "When I think about the road alone, I think of Sam. She came to therapy because she was in a relationship marked at times by mutual violence. Although I encouraged couples therapy, she insisted on attending sessions alone. So we explored the road alone, together. Even in our first session, she asked, 'Is this cycle of violence ever going to stop? I don't know if I should—or even want to—continue this relationship. I really like him, but I'm also afraid of the escalations and what we might do to each other.' In the sessions that followed, we explored their interactions and the relational pattern in which she and her partner became entangled. As Sam gained insight into these dynamics, she began to feel more at peace—alongside growing courage and hope. One day, Sam came in and shared that there had been another serious incident of violence. Together, they had decided to end the relationship. She had mixed feelings about the decision but remained committed to it. In the sessions that followed, she continued to speak often about the relationship—what she missed, and what had been painful. Even then, we *returned to the three puzzle pieces*: A lot happened to you, but what were the relationship dynamics underneath? And what do these dynamics reveal about what you and your ex-partner were each carrying?"

Gradually, Sam began to see that she was a 'contact-seeker'—someone who overwhelmed her partner with closeness, which made him feel suffocated and compelled him to push her away to regain space. She traced this pattern back to her early life as the daughter of a depressed mother. Sam had tried so hard to care for her mother, yet never saw any light in her mother's eyes when they looked at each other. Her first long-term relationship had been with a partner who buried himself in work. Even when he was physically present, he was emotionally unavailable—too exhausted for intimacy. Over time, Sam developed a deep fear that others wouldn't want to be with her, which led her to begin *claiming* her space in relationships.

Jef: "Some time later, Sam shared how making sense of the puzzle had helped her:

'Last week, I went on a date for the first time since the breakup. I was sitting across from a handsome man in a coffee shop. He listened to me attentively, and I found myself talking endlessly. I felt his presence in his engaged silence. And then, suddenly, it hit me: This is the same kind of partner again. Someone who is emotionally available, but who doesn't take up much space himself. I keep falling in love with the same kind of man.' 'I used to think I just fell for the wrong guys. But now I can see that I keep falling for men who offer the same kind of closeness. It meets a need I've carried since I was a little girl. These men do have light in their eyes when they look at me. But that very closeness also scares me. The moment they pull away—even slightly—I panic completely.' She told me how much it pleased her to finally see the puzzle so clearly. Where she had previously felt helplessly caught in a dynamic she didn't understand, she now felt like an active participant. That shift reduced her fear considerably and gave her *space to approach both this new relationship and her own emotions differently.*"

The wrong partner?

Sam's story shows us that the path we walk alone need not be so different from the one we walk together: both are journeys toward a deeper understanding of the self, the other, and the relationship. This makes sense—even though, at times, the growth gained may serve the next relationship rather than the current one, as is the case with Sam. Through exploration and learning to see things differently, new meanings can emerge. In this way, "the wrong partner" can unexpectedly become a familiar—and even the right—partner.

Lieven: "I always struggle with the phrase 'the wrong partner' and how often it's used. That doesn't align with what Sam is discovering here. In fact, she's saying, 'I'm falling for the right partner! *I fall for partners who might offer me something I deeply need.*' She won't fall for cold, self-absorbed men. That kind of partner wouldn't suit her. But when she meets an emotionally available man who pays attention to her, something shifts. Even from a slight distance, she starts to panic: 'See? He's going to leave too. I must not be worth much after all!' Then something intense and controlling awakens in Sam, and these men begin to shift—from 'quiet but available' to 'absent and unattainable.' They sense her fear that it's all going wrong again, just as they were trying their best. That's often when their own histories are triggered, too. The moment Sam realizes she has a good instinct for which men she needs—men who see her, who want to be there for her, but who will also sometimes say, 'Not right now, I need some space for myself'—and that this doesn't diminish their love or commitment, she'll be free to enter a relationship with closeness, but without overwhelming intensity. And in doing so, she's far more likely to receive the kind of commitment she's been seeking all along."

The story we tell ourselves—"I always fall for the wrong partner"—often reveals something about our self-image. It carries an underlying belief that there is something inherently wrong with us. In this way, it says little about the actual person in front of us: their qualities, their value, or whether they might be the right partner. The phrase is often confused with moral judgments about "good" or "bad" partners, shaped by societal norms. But that is another conversation entirely.

The fear or belief that we always choose the wrong partner can create the illusion that everything is predetermined. Sam's story, however, demonstrates two crucial things. First, that our intuition holds valuable insights—after all, we're drawn to certain types of partners because they promise something we deeply need. Second, it shows how a shared understanding of self, other, and relationship opens up new possibilities. These insights can lead to different patterns of interaction, making it more likely that the promise we sensed can actually be fulfilled.

There is nothing inherently wrong with you, or with the choice you made. What often goes wrong lies in the interaction cycle itself. That cycle can turn us into different partners than we were at the beginning. This is where the original promise we held for one another gets lost. But if we change the way we engage in that cycle, we can rediscover and transform that promise into something real—something no longer ruled by fear.

Conclusion: we can fight more lovingly

How strange and frightening it can be to love someone deeply, to want nothing more than to avoid escalating conflict or hurting one another… and yet, it happens anyway. In hindsight, it often feels incomprehensible. You may not recognize yourself or your partner in those moments, and you often can't even recall how it all began. All you know is that you never want it to happen again. So you start fighting just to avoid ending up in that place.

Some people are fortunate enough that these painful experiences actually shake them awake. They see each other more clearly, reconnect, and grow closer. But for many others, conflict creates a lingering fog between them and their partner. It may feel like a wall, a pane of glass, a swamp, or a maze. People describe it in many ways, but the common thread is a sense of disconnection—they just can't reach each other. There may be a period of peace, but something still feels unbridgeable. For these couples, it can be profoundly helpful to piece together—often with outside—support—the puzzle of their relationship: to understand each other's inner worlds and outward behaviors, the stories that shape them, and the way all these elements interact to pull them into a destructive cycle. This work honors their love and the effort they've already invested. It takes time and space to understand these dynamics and, when possible, to share them with each other. This process is not just engaging or insightful—it's transformative. By understanding the cycle and the puzzle pieces, couples can learn to relate to each other differently, and together create space for what they truly need.

Sometimes this work can be done together, within the current relationship. Sometimes it must happen separately, in reflection and healing apart from the partner. Sometimes the violence or harmful patterns stop temporarily, and sometimes they end completely. And sometimes this shared effort enables couples to learn how to fight more lovingly with each other—or, in some cases, to part with care and allow a future relationship to benefit from what they've learned.

However the road unfolds, we hope your search for safe, vibrant love continues. It's a journey you don't have to walk alone—on the contrary, it's one that connects you to many others. In doing this work, you're not only offering a gift to yourself but also to those around you.

We want to leave you with three gifts for anyone undertaking this quest for a safer relationship:

the gift of time, the gift of trust, and the gift of courage. Facing painful escalations with your partner is never easy. Looking directly at the harm you've caused—or endured—can be overwhelming. Revealing the vulnerable inner experiences beneath those reactions can feel frighteningly raw. Listening to your partner's vulnerability may stir pain you'd rather avoid. It takes immense time, trust, and courage to engage in this process—and to stay with it. We offer you these gifts with open hands. And by the way: if you've made it this far in the book, you've already given yourself the gift of time. You've already shown courage by being willing to look at yourself and your interactions honestly. We hope this book has helped you feel, even a little more, that a way out of these painful patterns is possible. Let this be the beginning of something.

We've witnessed hundreds of couples do this work before you, and there will be many more after you. Learning to fight more lovingly is not easy. It involves effort, vulnerability, sweat, and sometimes pain. But we also know it can bring emotional depth, tenderness, and connection—the kind you may not have dared to hope for in a long time. We are most certainly cheering you on from the sidelines.

Reflect and relate

Take a moment to pause and connect these ideas to your own experience.

Endings can take many forms—a pause after a fight, a shared realization, or the decision to walk separate paths. These questions invite you to reflect on what "ending" might mean in your own life, and how awareness can become part of healing.

1. When you ask yourself, "Will this fight ever end?", what are you truly longing for—peace, safety, connection, understanding, …?

2. How do you and your partner (or ex-partner) each try to stop escalation? Did you ever value your partner for this attempt?

3. Imagine being able to say to your partner, calmly: "I don't want to hurt you, I just want this to stop." How important would it be for your relationship to say this aloud?

4. Have you ever experienced a "relapse"—a return to escalation after things seemed better? If you take a close look at your experience, what does it tell about the feelings or longings that are still unresolved?

5. If you've chosen or considered walking the road alone, what helps you stay connected to what you've learned—about yourself, about love, about your position in a relationship, about what you need to feel safely connected?

To end this book, we invite you to a final reflection that captures the entire process of feeling and thinking you went through while reading:

What would it mean for you to "fight more lovingly"—with yourself, with your partner, or in future relationships?

Paint the picture and taste the words that accompany the image. How does it feel to imagine this and say this aloud to yourself, your partner or someone else that is important to you?

We hope this helps you feel that love is worth fighting for.

References

Aldarondo, E. (1996). Cessation and persistence of wife assault: A longitudinal analysis. *American Journal of Orthopsychiatry*, 66, 141–151.

Feld, S. L., & Strauss, M. A. (1989). Escalation and desistance of wife assault in marriage. *Criminology*, 27, 141–161.

Jasinski, J. L. (2001). Physical violence among Anglo, African American, and Hispanic couples: Ethnic differences in persistence and cessation. *Violence and Victims*, 16, 479–490.

Merchant, L.V., & Whiting, J. B. (2017). A grounded theory study of how couples desist from intimate partner violence. *Journal of Marital and Family Therapy*, 44, 590–605.

Index

www.ingramcontent.com/pod-product-compliance
Lightning Source LLC
LaVergne TN
LVHW010947110826
845149LV00015B/3244

* 9 7 8 1 0 4 1 1 6 1 7 3 8 *